THE PRIMARY MANAGEMENT OF MUSCULOSKELETAL TRAUMA

THE PRIMARY MANAGEMENT OF MUSCULOSKELETAL TRAUMA

David Seligson, MD
Professor and Vice Chair
Chief of the Fracture Service
Department of Orthopaedics
University of Louisville School of Medicine
Louisville, Kentucky

Kurt Voos, MD
Department of Orthopaedics
University of Louisville School of Medicine
Louisville, Kentucky

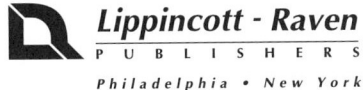

Lippincott - Raven
PUBLISHERS
Philadelphia • New York

Acquisitions Editor: Kathey Alexander
Developmental Editor: Emilie Linkins
Senior Production Editor: Virginia Barishek
Production Service: Tage Publishing Service
Compositor: Compset, Inc.
Printer/Binder: Maple Press
Cover Designer: Lou Fuiano
Cover Printer: Lehigh Press

Copyright ©1997 by Lippincott–Raven Publishers. All rights reserved. This book is protected by copyright. No part of it may be reproduced, stored in a retrieval system, or transmitted, in any form or by any means—electronic, mechanical, photocopy, recording, or otherwise—without the prior written consent of the publisher, except for brief quotations embodied in critical articles and reviews. Printed in The United States of America. For information write Lippincott–Raven Publishers, 227 East Washington Square, Philadelphia, PA 19106-3780.

Materials appearing in this book prepared by individuals as part of their official duties as U.S. Government employees are not covered by the above-mentioned copyright.

Library of Congress Cataloging-in-Publication Data
Seligson, David.
   The primary management of musculoskeletal trauma / David Seligson, Kurt Voos.
     p.   cm.
   Includes bibliographical references and index.
   ISBN 0-397-51389-5
   1. Fractures. 2. Joints—Wounds and injuries. I. Voos, Kurt.
  II. Title.
   [DNLM: 1. Fractures—therapy. 2. Bone and Bones—injuries.
  3. Soft Tissue Injuries—therapy. 4. Triage—methods. WE 175
  S465p 1997]
  RD101.S443   1997
  617.1'5—dc20
  DNLM/DLC
  for Library of Congress   96-42532
                                                                  CIP

Care has been taken to confirm the accuracy of the information presented and to describe generally accepted practices. However, the authors, editors, and publisher are not responsible for errors or omissions or for any consequences from application of the information in this book and make no warranty, express or implied, with respect to the contents of the publication.

    The authors, editors and publisher have exerted every effort to ensure that drug selection and dosage set forth in this text are in accordance with current recommendations and practice at the time of publication. However, in view of ongoing research, changes in government regulations, and the constant flow of information relating to drug therapy and drug reactions, the reader is urged to check the package insert for each drug for any change in indications and dosage and for added warnings and precautions. This is particularly important when the recommended agent is a new or infrequently employed drug.

    Some drugs and medical devices presented in this publication have Food and Drug Administration (FDA) clearance for limited use in restricted research settings. It is the responsibility of the health care provider to ascertain the FDA status of each drug or device planned for use in their clinical practice.

9 8 7 6 5 4 3 2 1

PREFACE

This book is a guide for medical students and other health professionals who see patients with skeletal trauma. It provides an introduction to clinical problems, a vocabulary about skeletal injury, and an indication of care routines for the triage of patients with acute musculoskeletal injury. *Triage* means sorting. This guide tells which patients can be discharged from an emergency room, which injuries require admission to a hospital, and which injuries need urgent specialty consultation. It is not meant to be authoritative, and it is not a replacement for judgment and common sense.

It is hard to learn about musculoskeletal injury on a short assigned rotation. One may want to examine a knee, make a short leg cast, put in a traction pin and thereby accomplish a basic menu of tasks.

Injuries present illogically. It takes time and experience to acquire skills in the evaluation and emergent care of skeletal injuries. Each case has a lesson for the thoughtful health care professional. An introductory book such as this one can help one to get oriented.

Fractures and sprains are the result of mechanical overload of bone and ligaments. Since no two injuries are exactly alike and no two patients are exactly the same, each injury is unique, having many possible solutions for treatment. The authors wish to emphasize that there is no "accepted" or best way to care for broken bones and soft tissue injuries. There are patterns of injuries and alternatives in treatment.

Injuries to the musculoskeletal system are of major socioeconomic importance. This guide to their triage is presented with the hope that it will improve communication about the care of musculoskeletal trauma.

DAVID SELIGSON, MD
KURT VOOS, MD

CONTENTS

PART I ■ GENERAL PRINCIPLES 1

1. Orthopedic Terminology 1
2. History, Examination, and Investigation 7
3. An Approach to Evaluating Skeletal X-rays for Injury 9
4. Polytrauma: The Patient with Multiple Injuries 13
5. The Open Fracture 17
6. Fracture Emergencies 23
7. The Treatment of Musculoskeletal Injury—An Overview 27
8. – – – itis and Other Diagnoses 33
9. Splints and Casts 37
10. Pain 43
11. Orthopedic Instrumentation 47
12. Traction and Suspension 53
13. Legal and Economic Aspects of Musculoskeletal Injury 57

PART II ■ REGIONAL INJURIES 61

14. Fractures and Dislocations about the Shoulder 63

15 Fractures of the Humerus Shaft   69
16 Elbow Injuries   77
17 Forearm Fractures   83
18 Wrist Injuries   87
19 Hand Fractures and Soft Tissue Injuries   95
    A. Hand Fractures   96
    B. Soft Tissue Injuries of the Hand   97
20 Pelvic and Acetabulur Fractures   103
21 Hip Fractures and Dislocations   109
    A. Hip Fractures   110
    B. Hip Dislocations   117
22 Femoral Shaft Fractures   119
23 Injuries about the Knee   123
    A. Knee Injuries   123
    B. Fractures of the Distal Femur and Proximal Tibia   124
    C. Patella Fractures   129
    D. Ligamentous Injuries of the Knee and Knee Dislocations   131
24 Leg Fractures   139
25 Ankle Injuries   145
    A. Ankle Sprains   145
    B. Ankle Fractures   146
    C. Pilon Fractures   151
26 Foot Fractures   155
    A. Fractures and Dislocations of the Talus and Calcaneus   157
    B. Forefoot Fractures and Dislocations   158

27 Spine Fractures   163
    A. Cervical Spine Fractures and Dislocations   166
    B. Thoracolumbar Fractures   171
    C. Acute Low Back Pain   174

PART III ■ CASE HISTORIES AND SELF-TEST   179

Suggested Readings   229

Index   235

PART I
GENERAL PRINCIPLES

Chapter 1
Orthopedic Terminology

Language is a means of communication. The following glossary explains terms that are in common use among musculoskeletal traumatologists. These terms are not necessarily logical. If one knows what an abbreviation means, then more of what is happening to injured patients will be understandable:

avascular necrosis—death of bone from lack of blood supply; osteonecrosis

Barton's fracture—a fracture of the distal radius in which the dorsal articular margin of the radius is displaced

boxer's fracture—an impacted fracture where the head of the fifth metacarpal is driven into its neck

burst fracture—a fracture of a vertebral body, usually the result of axial loading; bone fragments may be pushed into the spinal canal

chance (slice) fracture—a fracture of a thoracic or lumbar vertebra, often the result of wearing a seat belt, in which the fracture line extends from the spinous process through the pedicles, and then through the vertebral body in an anterior to posterior direction; an unstable injury

closed—not open; the fracture does not communicate with the atmosphere

Colles' fracture—a general term used for all distal radius fractures that are dorsally displaced

comminuted—splintered, many pieces

compound—the break communicates with the atmosphere

compression fracture—a fracture caused by axial overload of bone, commonly seen in the spine and the calcaneus

dislocation—a bone pulled out of joint

ExFix—external fixateur—a system of pins drilled into bone and held together by clamps and rods to stabilize a bone or joint

Galeazzi's fracture—a fracture of the distal radius with dislocation of the distal ulna

green stick fracture—a pediatric fracture where one cortex is fractured and the other is bent but not fractured

hangman's fracture—a fracture of the C2 vertebra in which both pedicles are fractured, usually the result of a hyperextension injury

Jefferson's fracture—a burst fracture of the atlas, usually the result of axial compression

Jones' fracture—an avulsion fracture of the proximal diaphysis of the fifth metatarsal

LAC—long arm cast—a cast immobilizing the elbow and wrist

Lisfranc's fracture-dislocation—fracture-dislocation of the tarsometatarsal joint

LLC—long leg cast (above the knee)

Malgaigne's fracture—an unstable fracture of the pelvis in which there is both an anterior and posterior fracture in the pelvic ring

mallet finger—a finger deformity where the extensor mechanism is injured; may be associated with a fracture of the distal phalanx

malunion—a fracture healed in a deformed position

meniscectomy—excision of a meniscus of the knee; may either be partial (partial meniscectomy) or complete

Monteggia's fracture—a fracture of the proximal ulna with dislocation of the radial head

nonunion—the failure or inevitable failure of fracture healing to occur (generally longer than one year)

NWB—non-weight-bearing

open—communicating with the atmosphere (a synonym for compound)

ORIF—open reduction internal fixation— surgically expose a fracture, align the bone, and hold it in place with plate, screws, or wires

Osgood-Schlatter's disease—painful swelling of the tibial tubercle in a youth

osteosynthesis—the operative stabilization of a broken bone with an appliance—plate, nail, or fixateur

parry fracture (night-stick fracture)—an isolated fracture of the ulna shaft

pathologic fracture—a break through diseased bone

Phalen's test—pain at the median nerve at the wrist when the wrist is placed in volar flexion

pilon fracture—fracture into the weight-bearing distal tibia articular surface

pseudoarthrosis—an unhealed bone; literally a false joint (a synonym for nonunion)

POP—plaster-of-Paris

PWB—partial-weight-bearing

ROM—range of motion

reduce—set, put into position

SAC—short arm cast

Segond's fracture—avulsion fracture of the knee joint capsule from the lateral aspect of the proximal tibia; high association with anterior cruciate ligament injuries

simple fracture—not splintered; a clean break

SLC—short leg cast (below the knee)

Smith's fracture (reverse Colles' fracture)—a volarly displaced distal radius fracture

spondylosis—arthritic changes in spinal joints, e.g., spurs and disc space narrowing

spondylolisthesis—translation of the more superior vertebral body in an anterior direction on the inferior vertebral body (if condition is reversed, this is termed retrolisthesis)

sprain—a torn ligament or joint capsule

strain—a torn muscle–tendon unit

straddle fracture—pelvic fracture in which there are fractures of bilateral superior and inferior pubic rami

tendinitis—inflammation of a tendon

tenosynovitis—inflammation of a tendon sheath

torus fracture (greenstick or buckle fracture)—fracture of only one cortex; usually seen in children

valgus—turned out of a circle drawn around the body; e.g., knock-knees = genu valgus

varus—turned in to a circle drawn around the body; e.g., bow legs = genu varus

Volkmann's ischemic contracture—end result of compartment syndrome in which there is contracture, fibrosis, and muscle atrophy; high association with supracondylar humerus fractures

WBAT—weight bearing as tolerated

Chapter 2

History, Examination, and Investigation

Musculoskeletal injury such as bruises, torn ligaments, and broken bones can be caused by a simple fall, sports activities, and auto accidents. Its spectrum varies from life-threatening, polytrauma injury to a subtle disruption of the stability of the knee. Often it is difficult to put together the story, the physical findings, and the results of diagnostic tests until days after the accident. The diagnostic clues are not always obvious. Pain and swelling are not necessarily present immediately after the event; it may take several days for them to appear. For example, a patient with a severe bruise on the forehead after a car accident may not initially have neck pain. The story, however, suggests the possibility of whiplash, and cervical spine films should be included as part of the workup. X-ray is indispensable to evaluation of any injury, however, an x-ray is only one dimension for assessment of skeletal injury. Signs of acutely torn ligaments on x-rays may be subtle. It is here that the physical examination is important. The examination is directed by the complaint, the history, and radiographic findings.

SITUATION + EXAMINATION + X-RAY = DIAGNOSIS

(Remember the three components of orthopedic problem solving: **SEX** = situation, evaluation, x-ray). For example, after a motor vehicle accident a front seat passenger complains of a sore knee. X-rays are taken in the emergency room. The x-rays are normal. Now the examiner places varus and valgus forces to evaluate the medial and lateral collateral ligaments, respectively.

Similarly, the cruciate ligaments are tested by the anterior and posterior drawer tests. Examination is not guided by the patient's assessment of pain. Slightly separated ligaments may actually be more painful than completely torn ones. In stressing a knee the examiner must determine if the ligament is damaged, but functionally intact (**grade I sprain**), if the joint opens a little because the ligament is partially torn (**grade II sprain**), or if the completely torn ligament offers no resistance to stress (**grade III sprain**) (See Table 2-1).

For some patients, the injury is too painful to allow an adequate examination. Then an anesthetic may be required to evaluate the injury. The patient is splinted and arrangements made with a specialist to reevaluate the condition. The examination under anesthesia can be performed in outpatient surgery.

A limb with fractures should be splinted to avoid pain and further damage. The assessment of the peripheral pulses and function of major nerves is carefully recorded. It is important to be aware of patterns of injury, typical stories, and special associations. For example, fractures of the femoral shaft have a high incidence of femoral neck fractures; patients who fall from ladders and roofs sustain fractures to the lumbar spine and calcaneus. Painful wrist tendinitis, **DeQuervain's disease**, is commonly associated with pregnancy and delivery.

TABLE 2-1 Grading of Sprains

GRADE		LIGAMENT DAMAGE
I	**Mild**	Ligament functionally intact
II	**Moderate**	Ligament is partially torn
III	**Severe**	Ligament is completely torn (offers no resistance to stress)

Chapter 3

An Approach to Evaluating Skeletal X-rays for Injury

1. Catalog the x-rays. How many views do you have? Are they the ones you need to evaluate the problem? Do you have the correct films? Are they labeled with the patient's name and the date taken? Is there an **R** or **L** marker on each film?
2. Inspect the soft tissue. Muscle plane of the body should be smooth, continuous lines. When both sides are on the film, the lines should be symmetrical. Attempt to identify the presence of air or swelling. The presence of air would indicate communication with the environment and thus an open injury. Soft tissue swelling—an increase in the distance between the surface of a limb and the bone—indicates injury.
3. Inspect the bone. Is bone density normal, increased, or decreased? Are generalized skeletal abnormalities present, such as dysplasia, cysts, exostosis? Follow the cortical margins of each bone in the x-ray, looking for breaks in the cortex. Follow fracture lines as they traverse the skeleton. Fractures are angular, jagged, sharp discontinuities.
4. Describe the location of the fracture(s) with respect to either the proximal one-third, middle one-third, or distal one-third of the bone or as diaphyseal, metaphyseal, or

involving the growth plate. Next describe the fracture pattern (Figure 3-1) (spiral, oblique, or transverse) and complexity (simple, comminuted, or complex). Describe angulation (e.g., there appears to be approximately 30° of angulation with the apex directed posteriorly).

5. Next describe apposition (i.e., the degree to which the two bone ends contact each other). The distal fragment should be described with respect to the proximal fragment (e.g., the distal fragment appears to be displaced approximately 25% medial to the proximal fragment).

6. Look at each joint. Is the joint space normal or narrow? Are arthritic findings such as osteophytes present? Look for the presence of air, fluid levels, and a fat-pad sign. Fluid in a joint elevates the periarticular fat pad away from the surface of the cortex. A possible fat-pad sign indicates the presence of effusion. Do fractures involve the joint? Is the joint surface smooth, or are there areas of depression? Is joint alignment correct relative to the joints above and below?

More is not always better. Not every neck pain needs a CT, and not every back injury merits an MRI. It is vital to form a concept about the potential extent of the injury and set a sensible plan for care. The patient with normal cervical alignment will be taken care of in an outpatient setting, and the patient with a burst fracture will need inpatient specialty care. Neither requires a long stay for diagnostic imaging in the emergency room.

Finally, remember that an x-ray is a black and white snapshot of anatomy. It contains a tremendous amount of information, if you learn what to look for.

FIGURE 3-1 Diaphyseal fracture types. The basic fracture patterns are seen. Properly identify the fracture type so that it can accurately be described to the treating physician.

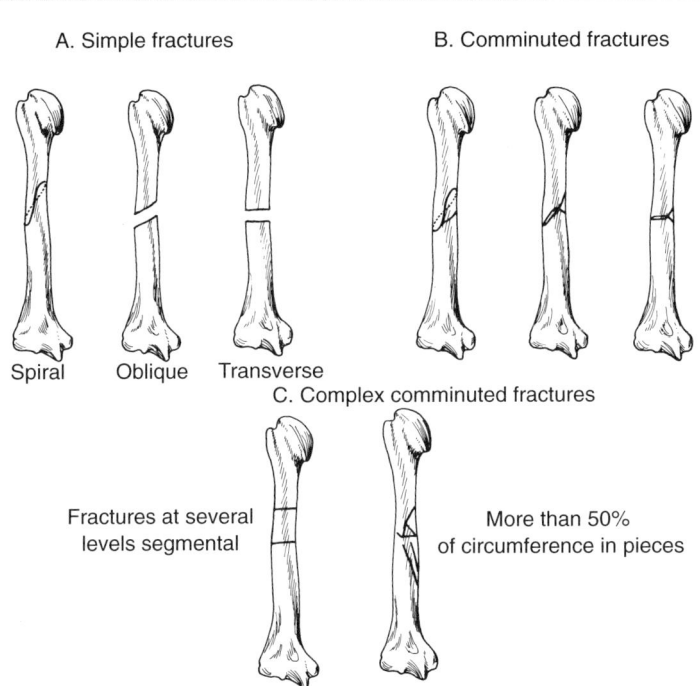

Chapter 4
Polytrauma: The Patient with Multiple Injuries

A polytrauma patient is one who has severe injury to multiple organ systems—for example, closed head injury, rupture of the spleen, and fractured femur all in the same patient. The diagnosis and treatment of the musculoskeletal injuries has a lower priority than life-saving measures such as the placement of a chest tube to drain a hemopneumothorax. Nonetheless, assessing, stabilizing and planning for the care of broken bones is best done along with the measures that must be taken to stabilize the high-priority organ systems. If a C.T. of the head is required to rule out subdural hematoma, there is usually enough time to splint the patient's fractured tibia prior to obtaining the head scan. Similarly, a pin for skeletal traction can be inserted while the fluid for a diagnostic peritoneal lavage is running in or out. The severity of the problem directs the workup. Multiple x-rays of a complex tibial pilon fracture are inappropriate in a patient with a liver laceration and hemodynamic instability. Remember that the **D**'s and **F**'s (**dislocations** and **fractures**) of trauma care follow the **ABC**'s (**airway, breathing, circulation**).

Some features of musculoskeletal injuries become particularly important in polytrauma patients. The presence of pain and deformity is generally helpful in identifying injury; its absence is not. In fact, even a displaced fracture may initially not be painful to manipulate. The examiner's assessment on inspection, palpation, and range-of-motion testing is useful. Notice whether the limb is straight; appreciate subcutaneous crepitus from a fracture; ascertain ligamentous instability at a joint. However, there is nothing to be learned from handling a limb in which the injury is visually evident. The next steps are an x-ray and planned treatment. The physical examination of the musculoskeletal system in polytrauma is not primarily an interaction with the patient. One moves a limb not to obtain the patient's response but rather to see whether the restraining ligaments are functioning normally. It is the examiner's assessment that helps in diagnosis.

The minimum workup of the severely injured patient, conscious or not, includes a lateral x-ray of the cervical spine and a flat plate of the pelvis, as well as palpation of the shoulders, elbows, hips, and knees. In the conscious patient neurologic function in the arms and legs is quickly checked by testing grip strength in the hands ("squeeze my hands") and measuring the ability to plantarflex the feet against resistance ("step on the gas"). Note that it is not crucial to detect all minor injuries to the acral skeleton, such as a nondisplaced medial malleolus fracture or a thumb sprain, but it is important not to miss the diagnosis of an unstable spine fracture or a hip dislocation. Ultimately, since each injury is unique, the judgment of how a lesion will behave depends on the passage of time.

Survival in the severely injured is improved by making the skeleton stable. A variety of strategies are available, including intramedullary nailing, external fixation, and screwplate fixation. Collectively these operative methods for holding bones in place are called *osteosynthesis* (*osteo* = bone and *synthesis* = putting together). Nonoperative methods of fracture care include casting, bracing, and traction. In multiple trauma, more active surgical treatment may be advisable, because the cardiopulmonary dynamics improve considerably when the patient can be mobilized at least to a sitting position as a consequence of fracture fixation.

The severity of injury to an individual can be quickly estimated by applying a number from one to five, the abbreviated injury scale (AIS), for each of the three most severely injured systems. One, two, and three points are given for mild, moderate, and severe injuries, respectively. Four points are given for a potentially lethal injury with a usually successful outcome (e.g., tension pneumothorax) and five points for a usually lethal outcome (e.g., ruptured aorta). Simple fractures are given two (moderate) points. The sum of the squares of the values given to the most severely injured systems is the injury severity score (**ISS**). For example, a patient with a ruptured spleen (4), fractured femur (2), and transient loss of consciousness (1) has an ISS of 21.

$$4^2 + 2^2 + 1^2 = 21$$

The ISS ranges between 1 and 75. In general, polytrauma means an injury severity score of greater than 20. Approximately one-half of the patients with an ISS greater than 35 will not survive. Age of greater than 50 years worsens the prognosis two-fold (see Table 4-1).

TABLE 4-1 The Injury Severity Score

Systems:	Cardiopulmonary	
	Central nervous	
	Gastrointestinal	
	Genitourinary	
	Musculoskeletal	
Abbreviated Injury Score (AIS):	Mild	1
	Moderate	2
	Severe	3
	Lethal	4
	Death	5

$$\text{ISS} = \mathbf{A}^2 + \mathbf{B}^2 + \mathbf{C}^2$$

Where **A, B,** and **C** are the three most injured systems.

Chapter 5

The Open Fracture

A fracture is defined as **open** or **compound** when the fracture site communicates with the outside atmosphere. All open fractures require urgent treatment. Do not reduce a grossly contaminated open fracture, as this may cause further contamination by infolding foreign material into the wound. To control infection the wound must be enlarged, the bone inspected and cleansed (i.e., débrided), the fracture stabilized, and antibiotic therapy initiated. Triple antibiotic therapy is usually started in the emergency room, one good program includes Kefzol, Tobramycin, and penicillin.

Wound debridement should take place in an operating room where conditions are optimal. An operating room is a clean area with good lights and instruments. Positioning the patient and preparing the skin are part of the usual routine! The sterility of the instruments is checked. Priorities in the treatment of compound fractures include assessment and definitive care of other injuries such as pneumothorax, ruptured spleen, etc. and the mobilization of appropriate resources for the operative care of the fracture. It has not been shown that the immediate administration of antibiotics is helpful nor that precipitous operative intervention achieves results. However, delays beyond eight hours probably do increase the risk of infection.

In addition to the usual general preparation for an operation—CBC, type and cross-matched blood, chest x-ray, EKG, and urine analysis—the patient should have an x-ray of the fracture, temporary splinting, and a clean dressing (for example, providoneiodine-soaked 4 × 4 gauze pads) applied to the wound. Repeated inspection of the injury under nonsterile conditions can lead to limb-threatening wound infection. Report the size of the wound of compounding as grade I, II, or III, depending on whether it is a small puncture (less than 1 inch), moderate, or large (more than 4 inches), note whether bone or tissue is lost, and assess the function of major nerves and blood vessels. Even when marked contamination is present, traction for splinting may be helpful in restoring circulation to a compromised limb.

Injuries that cause a communication between viscera and bone, such as a gunshot wound to the abdomen with penetration of the colon and the iliac bone, are particularly sinister, since the contamination is difficult to extirpate. Inspect the back and buttocks of a patient with a ventral entrance wound to avoid missing this injury.

Traumatic amputations are a special case of compound fracture (Figures 5-1 through 5-3). Except for toe and finger amputations, which can be debrided and even skin-grafted in the emergency room, amputations all require operative inspection to create a clean wound, ligate vessels, and plan for closure and/or coverage.

With open-compound fractures remember to **ACT**:

Assess—circulation, nerve function, wound size, and x-rays

Cleanse—in an operating room, debride dead tissue and irrigate the wound

Treat—care for the skeletal injury, reconstruct torn structures, plan rehabilitation

FIGURE 5-1 In compound fractures, the bone may protrude through the skin.

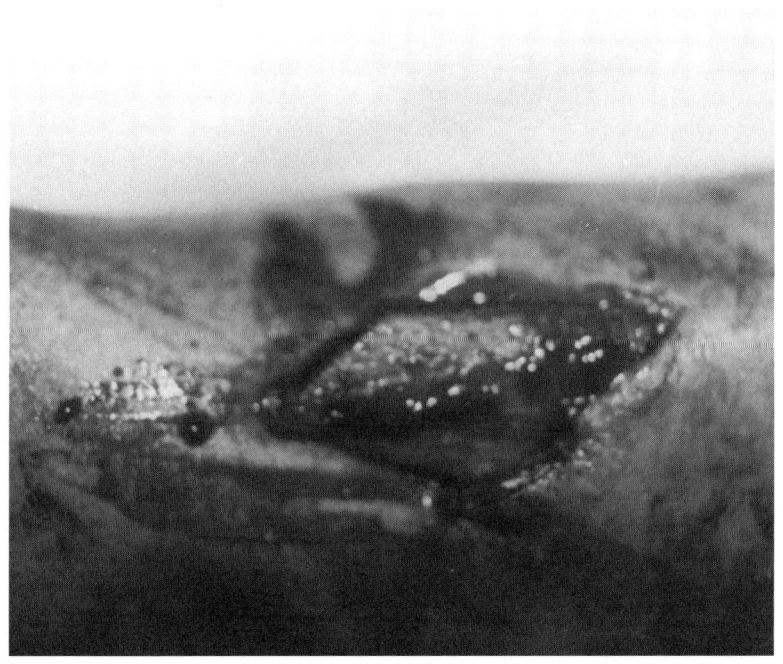

FIGURE 5-2 Debridement, reduction, and, in this case of a fractured tibia, external fixation were performed urgently in the operating room.

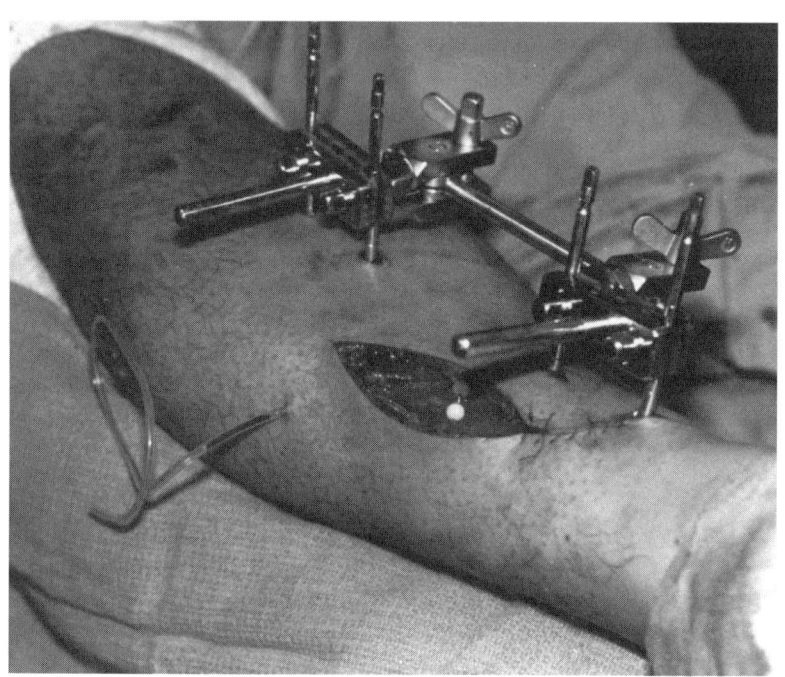

FIGURE 5-3 Multiple traumatic amputations from a woodsplitter injury. These and all traumatic amputations must be debrided and revised in the operating room.

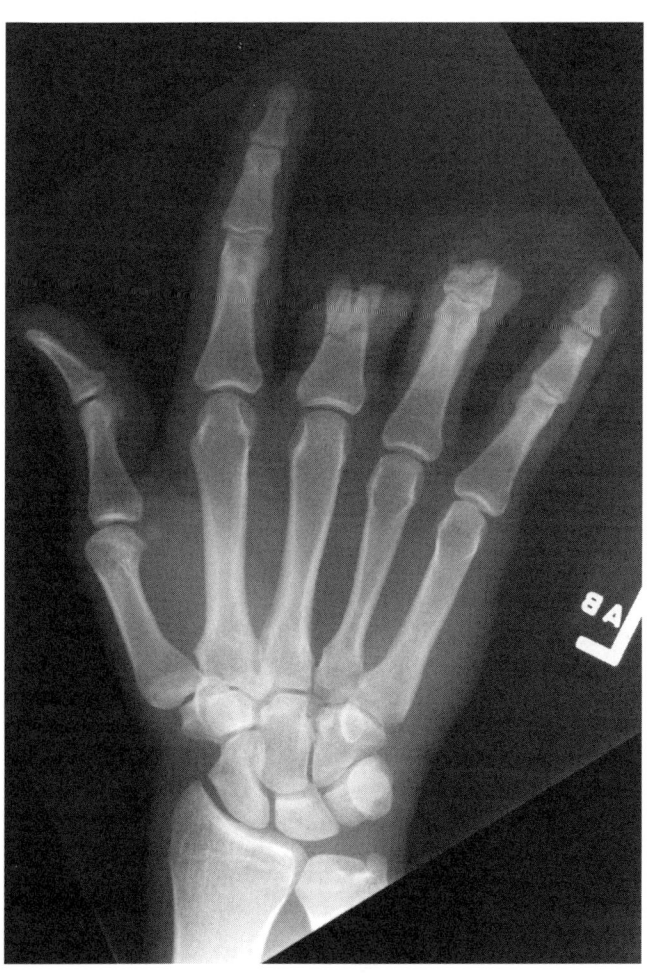

Chapter 6

Fracture Emergencies

In an emergency, immediate action is required to prevent permanent damage. Fracture emergencies take priority *after* the *ABC*'s of trauma care. (See Chapter 4.) Usually, the treatment of a closed or open fracture can be delayed. However, the following situations require rapid, decisive action.

1. UNREDUCED DISLOCATION OF A MAJOR JOINT

Diagnosis: Dislocation of the shoulder, elbow, hip, and knee is diagnosed clinically and verified radiologically (Figure 6-1).

Solution: Closed reduction; if necessary general anesthesia with transient muscle paralysis may be necessary to overcome muscle contractions and reduce the joint.

Complications: Delay in reduction increases the risk of osteonecrosis, nerve palsy, vascular compromise, or compartment syndrome

2. PROGRESSIVE LOSS OF NEUROLOGIC FUNCTION (SPINE OR EXTREMITY)

Diagnosis: When a reliable observer notes voluntary motor function (e.g., ability to dorsiflex the foot) that then is lost

Solution: Operative exploration—decompression, stabilization

FIGURE 6-1   Acute dislocation of the elbow. Note the fracture fragments in the prereduction film. This is not just an oblique film. The shaft of the radius does not line up with the capitellum. After closed reduction, the patient will need admission and possible surgery.

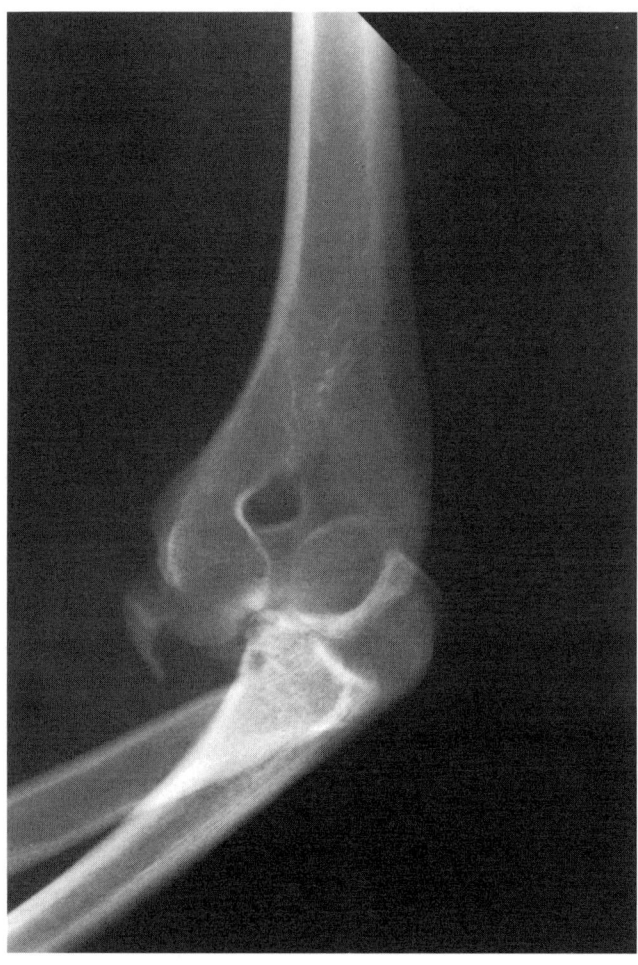

Complications: Irretrievable loss of neurologic function

3. PROGRESSIVE PAIN, PARALYSIS, PALLOR, AND PULSELESSNESS IN A LIMB (COMPARTMENT SYNDROME)

Obstruction of blood flow in a closed space, such as the muscular compartment of the leg, causes irrevocable death of muscle and loss of limb function.

Solution: Operative release of fascial compartments

Complications: Ischemic contracture

4. LACK OF CIRCULATION

Arteries and veins can be severed in penetrating injuries, lacerated by sharp edges of bone, or compressed from without or within.

Solution: Arteriography, exploration—revascularization

Complications: Failure to act leads to permanent loss of limb function, stiff joints, intractable pain or possible amputation. Prompt action can lead to normal function.

Chapter 7

The Treatment of Musculoskeletal Injury—An Overview

Bone, muscle–tendon units, and ligaments heal slowly. In general, adult skin is functionally healed in one to two weeks, tendons and ligaments in six to eight weeks, and long bones, e.g., the tibia, in four months (Figure 7-1). Scar maturation and bone remodeling, however, may go on for years. Many people ask, "Is it true that my bone is stronger after it has united?" If the healing callus is thicker than the fractured bone, it will be stronger—at least for a while. Bone will eventually be remodeled back to normal caliber in the years after it has healed, and then its breaking strength will be normal (Figure. 7-2).

When a **bone** is fractured, a hematoma from the bleeding bone ends forms around the fracture site. The environment of the hematoma sets in motion the repair process. Capillaries grow into the clot. There is a proliferation of osteoblasts. When the bony fragments move relative to each other, a **callus** forms (usually within the first two weeks). A callus is the palpable firm swelling of healing tissue at the fracture site. The process of callus formation reduces interfragmental motion and allows bone to form. When there is virtually no interfragmental motion, as in a nondisplaced

28 General Principles

FIGURE 7-1 Healing times.

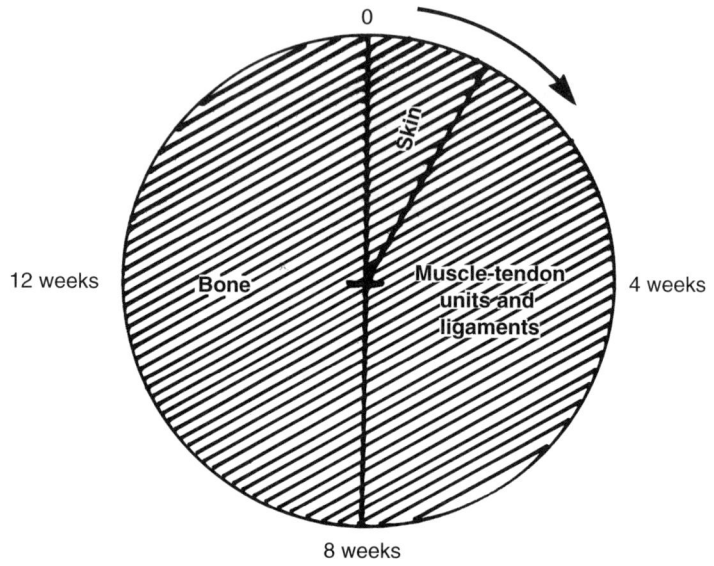

FIGURE 7-2 Not only did this motorcycle rider sustain a compound fracture, but the comminution of the tibia is severe (complex comminuted). Initial treatment was debridement and external fixation. Reconstruction will be difficult.

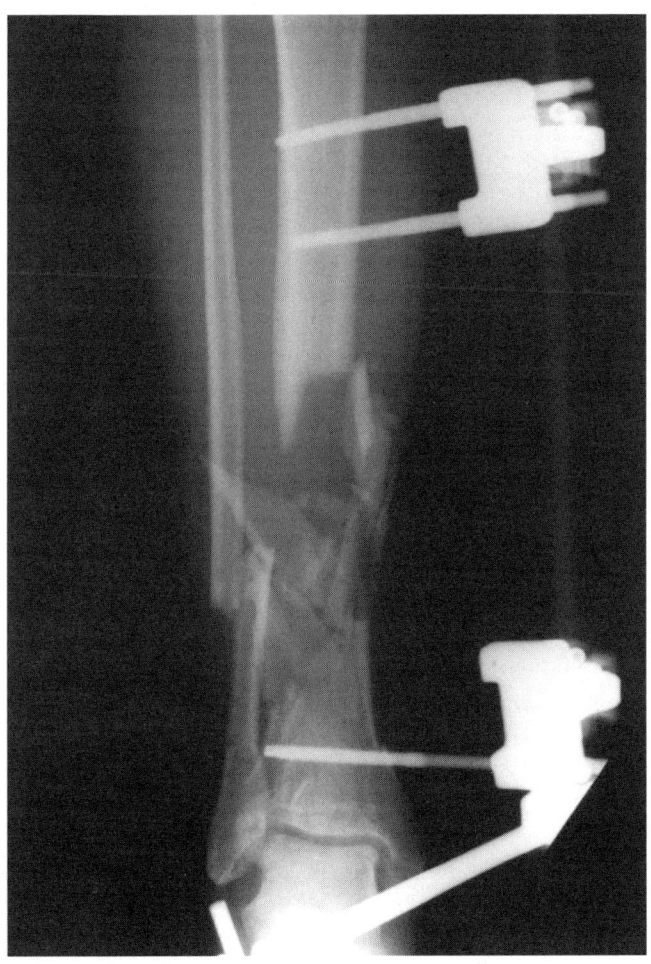

fracture, bone fragments remodel without callus. This is sometimes called **primary bone healing**, as compared with the formation of callus, which is **secondary bone healing**. Some plans for fracture treatment, such as the surgical placement of bone plates, screws, and nails, reduce interfragmental motion substantially, so that the fracture heals as if it were a nondisplaced fracture, i.e., it heals by primary bone healing. This procedure is an operative repair, as contrasted to using casts, traction, or braces to treat fracture, tendon or ligament injury. Nonoperative (sometimes called conservative) treatment with casts, traction, braces, splints, etc. allows some motion between bone fragments, and bone healing under these conditions occurs with callus formation. In reality, fractures whether treated operatively or nonoperatively have areas of contact healing and areas of callus formation. Bone remodeling is a continual process and is not complete until the reformation of the intramedullary canal. This process is dependent upon stresses that are placed upon the bone. Patients need to be told from their first visit with health care providers that repair of the skeleton is an active process in which they must participate.

Tendon repairs are made by both fibroblasts and macrophages. With tendon injuries in the hand it is important to immobilize the wrist and digits, as this leads to increased tendon strength and minimizes the chances of tendon rupture. However, the one disadvantage of immobilization is that it decreases range of motion, and physical and occupational therapy must then be employed to increase range of motion. It is possible to set up a dynamic splint that allows a healing tendon to move without putting it under load. Like the healing of bone, the strength of tendon repairs is time dependent (see Table 7-1).

The important thing to remember about **ligament** healing is that the ligament is weakened by immobilization. Mobilization results in improved range of motion and hypertrophy of the collagen fibril. In situations in which the ligament is completely disrupted, immobilization is required, unless the ligament is strongly reattached—for example, with a metal staple.

TABLE 7-1 Timetable for Healing of Tendons

7–14 days	weakest—disrupts with simple muscle pull
6–8 weeks	functionally healed—the muscle can move the tendon
6 months	maximum strength—returns toward normal tensile strength

In most situations the choice between an operative or a nonoperative (i.e., conservative treatment) strategy is clear. For example, a displaced intraarticular fracture that involves deformity of the articular surface requires operative treatment to minimize the complication of arthritis, which can significantly decrease range of motion and lead to the onset of chronic pain. However, in many circumstances different treatment approaches will provide equivalent results.

The risk-benefit equation is determined by the patient, the constellation of injuries, the available equipment and the physician's experience. In the initial triage of an injured patient, it may be best to leave alternatives open, since the pattern of care depends on expert evaluation of the exact nature of the injury (an assessment of the patient) and a considered selection of a treatment option.

Chapter 8

– – – itis and Other Diagnoses

The fundamental response of the body to injury is inflammation, which consists of the recruitment of leukocytes, the release of local tissue mediators, and alteration in vascularity in preparation for repair. In addition to inflammation, the diagnoses applicable to this process include arthritis, tendinitis, bursitis, and fasciitis.

Inflammation involving a joint can manifest as local warmth, pain, erythema, effusion, and restricted motion. The findings are variably present. For example, in a knee inflamed by a gonococcal infection the fluid is easy to detect. By contrast, in gout the fluid in the first metatarsal phalangeal joint is less obvious. Distinguish between *arthritis,* which is an inflammatory response to infection, crystals, or disease, and *arthrosis,* which is a joint-space change caused by an unfavorable mechanical situation. For example, years after medial menisectomy of the knee, excessive mechanical pressure because of loss of the shock-absorbing effect of the medial meniscus causes joint-space narrowing, overgrowth of osteophytes, and may lead to painful effusion and loss of motion.

Hyaline cartilage is a specialized tissue that covers the surfaces of joints and forms the growing ends of long bones. Fibrocartilage fills in spaces in the skeleton, e.g., the costochondral junctions. Maintenance of the integrity of cartilage depends on cartilage cells, which are entombed in proteoglycan matrix. Disturbance of this balance by rapid growth, overuse, or injury leads to fragmentation of cartilage, which is a cause of pain and swelling. These conditions are known as *osteochondroses* (Table 8-1).

TABLE 8-1 Common Osteochondroses

CONDITION	NAME	PRESENTATION
Tibial tubercle apophysitis	Osgood-Schlatter's disease	Painful swelling of the tibial tubercle in adolescent boys
Capital femoral epiphysitis	Legg-Calvé-Perthes disease	Sore hip in a child
Calcaneal apophysitis	Siever's disease	Painful heel, prepubertal
Epiphysitis of the capitellum	Little Leaguer's elbow	Pain, loss of extension
Inflammation of the costochondral junction	Costochondritis	Sore chest wall, middle age
Inflammation of pubic symphysis	Pubic symphysitis	Women after childbirth

The biology of tendons is equally specialized. Tendons deliver the power of muscles to joints. They may traverse narrow canals and turn corners around bone prominences. When tendons or ligaments become worn and/or frayed, their exposed fibers can incite the precipitation of calcium salts. Inflammation of a tendon in its sheath causes pain and limits performance. Usual sites are the Achilles' tendon, the biceps tendon in its groove at the shoulder, and the common extensor tendon origin at the elbow. These conditions are diagnosed by finding local tenderness over the area, pain on resisted motion, and negative x-rays. Rest, ice packs, anti-inflammatory medication, and sometimes local injections of corticosteroids are used in treating these conditions.

Tendinitis with deposition of calcium salts can be an accumulative process. When tendons course through bursae, the calcific deposits can grow and erupt into the bursa. Anatomic sites favoring this disorder are the supraspinatus tendon in the subacromial bursa, the gluteus medius tendon in the trochanteric bursa, and the flexor carpi ulnaris at the wrist. These conditions are called **calcific tendinitis** and **bursitis**. They are all varieties of **peritendinitis calcarea**. In the acute phase the pain may be intense and the x-rays negative. Longstanding calcific deposits are identified in their characteristic locations by x-ray.

Chapter 9

Splints and Casts

Immobilization is fundamental to the care of musculoskeletal injury. Splinting reduces pain. This is important not only for humane care, but also so that informed consent for treatment can be obtained, and so that accurate neurologic observation can be carried out. Splinting can be urgent, temporizing, or definitive. *Urgent* immobilization during patient assessment reduces pain and prevents injury. Simple devices such as sandbags, malleable splints, and triangular bandages are often sufficient. Emergency medical technicians often use these devices for transport. An important task in the initial assessment of an injured extremity is to check the splint and be certain that it has been applied without causing pressure or circulatory compromise. Feel gently along the extremity and slip a finger under buckles and bandages to assure that they are not too tight. If a bandage prevents venous return but does not occlude arterial inflow, it will have a *venous tourniquet effect*. This accentuates bleeding and causes limb swelling. If a splint is removed for examination of the patient, it should be replaced, particularly when a limb is unstable. If a patient needs an arteriogram, a twisted leg should be positioned to prevent its rolling around, which would make the study suboptimal and would risk compounding of a fracture. Radiographs taken in roughly standard positions are better for diagnosis than oddly angled projections. This is particularly true around joints.

Temporary splints are applied after diagnosis and can be used either for patients who are hospitalized for treatment or for patients who are sent home. Basic arm and non-weight-bearing leg splints can be made as shown in Figure 9-1. The limb is wrapped in cast padding; 10 to 12 thicknesses of plaster

FIGURE 9-1 Extremity splinting. Schematic representation of splint application. *A.* The initial step is to apply 3 to 4 layers of cast padding smoothly and evenly, with extra padding around bony prominences such as the malleoli. *B.* Next the splint material is dipped. The warmer the water, the shorter the curing time of the splint material. The curing is an exothermic process, so be sure that the water is not too warm, to avoid burning the patient. *C.* Next apply the splint to the extremity, making sure it conforms properly and does not come in contact with the skin. Once the splint has been applied, take a bandage while the splint is still moldable and wrap the extremity.

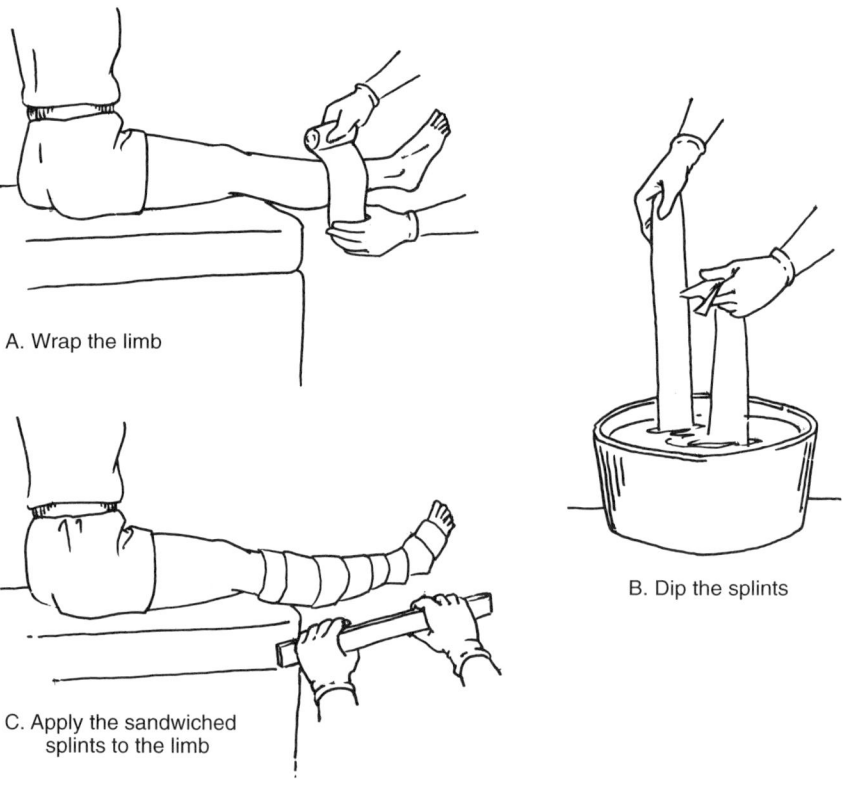

A. Wrap the limb

B. Dip the splints

C. Apply the sandwiched splints to the limb

the appropriate length are dipped in water; the plaster is sandwiched between layers of cast padding, fitted to the extremity and held in place with a loose bandage.

Splints are safe because they allow swelling. The cast-padding sandwich makes them easier to take off. Plaster with a covering of protective material is available in prefabricated rolls. Arm and leg splints are placed the full length of the limb, i.e., toe-to-calf or palm-to-forearm. Splints that stop in mid-arm or mid-leg can act as a fulcrum for diaphyseal fractures and can compromise circulation. Traditionally a limb is splinted in the "position of function." This position was used particularly for combat casualties. The thought was that, should circumstances delay further treatment, the stiff limb would be as functional as possible. In civilian practice specific injuries require splinting in the position most likely to result in good function. The hand is thus splinted with the metacarpal-phalangeal joints flexed and the web space maintained. Suggestions for splinting are found in the chapters on regional injuries (Part II).

Definitive treatment of most simple fractures can almost always be accomplished by splints. (Figure 9-2). Circular solid casts of plaster or fiberglass may be used, however, because they are more reliable in maintaining position. With a circular cast, the patient has more mobility, there is better control of pain and reduction, and the outer wrapping cannot come loose. However, casts are more dangerous than splints, because the limb can swell inside, causing circulatory compromise and tissue damage. A safe policy is not to send a patient home from the emergency room with a fresh injury in a circular cast unless the cast is *split* (The cast is cut medially and laterally and is spread, the padding is cut on one side to the skin, and then the cast is held in place with a loose wrap.) Splints will do the job with much less risk. Reduction can almost always be achieved again if it is lost. Tissue necrosis from a tight cast is irretrievable.

Circular casts for initial fracture treatment are applied over a layer of cast padding: hold the padding roll away from the limb and pull it gently so it conforms. Conversely, plaster-

FIGURE 9-2 The soft figure-of-eight splint for a clavicle fracture (note the buckles). In this child, emergency treatment is definitive treatment. At two weeks, reduction is maintained and there is early callus.

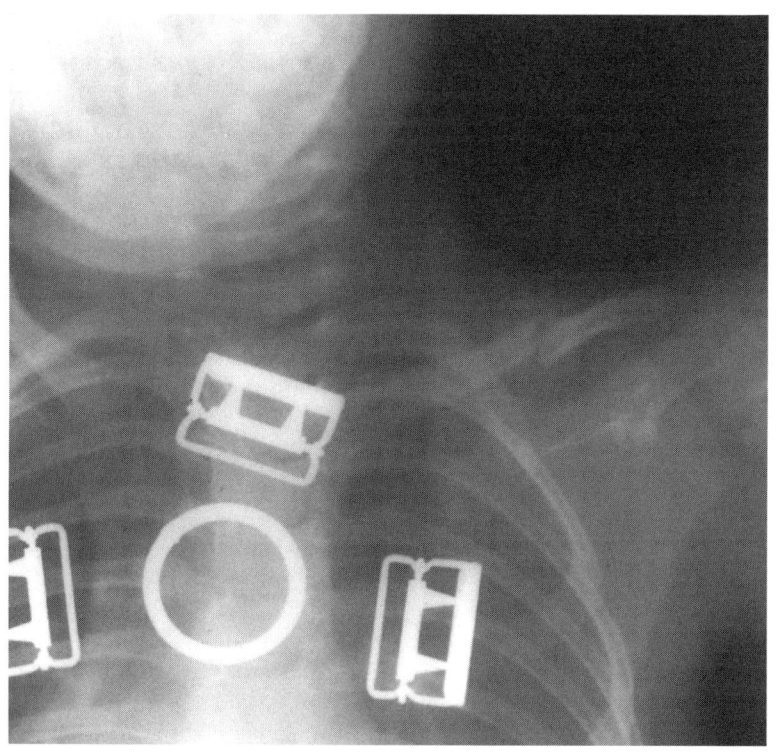

of-Paris is rolled close to the limb and "tucked" to make a smooth cast. The advantages and disadvantages of plaster of Paris and fiberglass circular casts are outlined in Tables 9-1 and 9-2. To learn to apply a good cast, seek out an experienced technician, work with that person, and keep trying. Casting is a real art.

TABLE 9-1 Plaster-of-Paris Casting

ADVANTAGES	DISADVANTAGES
Exact fit	Disintegrates when wet
Porous	Can burn the limb
Inexpensive	Messy

TABLE 9-2 Fiberglass Casting

ADVANTAGES	DISADVANTAGES
Light Weight	Not Porous
Water resistant	Hard to apply
Neat	Expensive

Chapter 10
Pain

Pain is a central nervous system phenomenon—an emotion: a usually unpleasant feeling that there is damage or dysfunction in a body part. Fractures and muscle-tendon injuries are painful! The amount of pain does not necessarily correlate with the extent of injury. A scarcely displaced acromioclavicular sprain (grade I) can be more painful than a fractured femur. The pain equation has many variables, which include temperature, time after injury, presence of shock, and emotional stability. Pain may be what brings the ambulatory patient to an emergency department. The severe polytrauma patient may seem to tolerate a great deal of invasive resuscitative procedures—intubation, chest tube, placement of skeletal traction—with minimal report of pain. However, if you ask the patient months later about recollections of initial care, the response may be the painful experience of a traction pin being placed. These memories never go away.

There are two fundamentally different types of pain. **Somatic** pain is carried centrally by myelinated, evolutionarily advanced axons with relatively few synapses. Somatic pain is specific, sharp, localized, epicritic pain. In contrast, **visceral** pain is a polysynaptic, vague, and poorly localized sensation. Remember, **S**omatic pain begins with **S** and is **S**pecific, while **V**isceral pain is **V**ague. An acute fracture produces sharp, localized pain at the site of injury. Irritation of a nerve root may, on the other hand, produce dull, burning, poorly localized discomfort (Table 10-1).

Somatic pain can be effectively managed locally by infiltration or nerve blocks and centrally with narcotics or narcotic equivalents. Visceral pain is more complex to treat because of its pervasive polysynaptic transmission. When visceral pain becomes chronic, it presents in specific syndromes such as

TABLE 10-1 Musculoskeletal Pain

TYPE	SOMATIC	VISCERAL
Quality	Sharp, knifelike, harmful	Dull, burning, annoying
Localization	Anatomic: along nerves or dermatomes	Poorly defined
Duration	Acute	Chronic
Cause	Injury	Irritation

phantom limb pain and the causalgias. These are notoriously difficult to control.

It is conceptually helpful to divide emergent care of musculoskeletal injury into three phases—evaluation, manipulation, and disposition. Interventions of different types for pain control have differing effectiveness and special rules for their use. In the treatment, for example, of a patient with a broken forearm, an extremely painful condition, intramuscular morphine may relieve pain but will prevent obtaining a valid consent for operative treatment. Understanding of triage facilitates humane treatment. There is no reason why an adult with an obviously broken arm should not receive a splint, and an x-ray, sign a consent, and get medication soon after entry into the emergency department.

During initial evaluation narcotic medications are not usually useful. They obtund the mind, depress vital functions, and mask physical findings. There are, however, a wide variety of orthopedic measures that can reduce pain. These include traction, splinting, use of ice, and positioning of the injured part. Even with a critically ill patient the routine should be to place sandbags around an unstable thigh with a possible hip or acetabulum fracture.

After diagnosis many injuries require some potentially painful manipulation. Here local anesthesia is the mainstay of pain management. Infiltration of the fracture hematoma reduces pain and facilitates reduction of a displaced distal radius fracture. A solution of 1% lidocaine without epinephrine is safe and short acting. Instillation of local anesthetic to the periosteum is a kind way to place a pin for skeletal traction.

In general, combinations of intravenous narcotics, barbiturates, and benzodiazepams do little more than reduce patient cooperation, increase awkwardness of procedures, and delay disposition. A possible exception is the use of a so-called 'lytic cocktail' for a pediatric patient. Sedative mixtures should be used with appropriate precautions. Vital signs are monitored during the procedure. A "crash cart" must be available. Continuous monitoring of oxygenation with a pulse oximeter is prudent. Two skilled professionals should be at the bedside. Anesthesia and fluoroscopy should be considered for managing difficult closed injuries in preference to moving a partially medicated patient back and forth for x-rays.

At the time of disposition, parenteral narcotics are useful for the patient who will be admitted to the hospital for treatment. Here small frequent doses of intravenous narcotics (e.g., morphine 2 mg I.V.) are appropriate. The homebound patient should be given a small amount of potent medication (e.g., codeine with aspirin) for severe injuries. Prescribing a nonsteroidal such as ibuprofen in the belief that narcotic abuse will flourish as a result of the appropriate and sparing use of effective medication for bona-fide injury is callous. The amount of medication should correspond to the instructions for scheduling a follow-up visit (Table 10-2).

TABLE 10-2 Pain Control for Injury

Evaluation	Mechanical measures	Splinting, evaluation, ice
Manipulation	Local measures	Infiltration, anesthesia, nerve blocks
Disposition	Systemic measures	Hospitalized—parenteral narcotics Home-bound—oral analgesics

Chapter 11

Orthopedic Instrumentation

The operative repair of displaced and intraarticular fractures is increasingly the norm. These procedures permit accurate reduction of fractures, decrease morbidity during healing, improve functional results, and decrease hospital stays. Fracture of the femur in an adult was previously managed with skeletal traction, followed by bracing. Hospitalization generally lasted two months. The incidence of deformity was considerable. Operative treatment has reduced the stay to a week and gives the patient a good result. Not only is the emergency department the point of initial contact for most patients with acute skeletal injury, but also patients often seek urgent care in the ER in the postoperative period. Broken bones are seldom planned, and treatment may occur far from home in a setting where follow-up is problematic. Hence, these postoperative patients may return to the ER with pain, drainage, and concern. The general function of the ER in postoperative patients is to expedite an arrangement for postoperative care rather than to comprehensively evaluate and solve the problem.

The three basic operative strategies for operative fracture care are intramedullary nails, plates and screws, and external fixateurs. Each has its own peculiar consequences. Intramedullary nails are metal tubes that are run lengthwise in the marrow cavity of long bones—most commonly the femur, tibia, and humerus—to stabilize fractures. Often the nails can be placed through a small incision at the end of the limb. The nails are finger-sized in diameter and run the length of the bone. Reduction and nail placement is performed under fluoroscopy. Screws can be inserted transversely through holes in the nails at either end (interlocking) to control length and rotation. Problems can include postoperative hematomas, loss of fixation, and thrombophlebitis. A change in the shape of the limb, significant increased swelling, appreciable drainage, or fever are indications to bring the patient into the hospital for observation under the care of a specialist. Mild temperature elevations (37°–38° C) and some increase of pain or swelling with increased activity are not unusual. Often there is enough serous drainage from a drain site to soak a 4 × 4 gauze pad. Send the patient home on a program of decreased activity and elevation with outpatient follow-up. Prescribe suppressive antibiotics such as an oral cephalosporin.

Plate-and-screw fixation is an accepted form of treatment for fractures, especially near joints and of the radius and ulna. This surgery is usually called **osteosynthesis.** It involves making an incision over the fracture, exposing the ends of the fracture, placing the fractured bone ends in an exact position, and then holding the position with a metal plate affixed with screws (**ORIF**). (See Figure 11-1.) These operations are most commonly used for the treatment of ankle fractures, where the plate is used on the fibula, for tibial plateau fractures, where the plate is used to hold the proximal tibia together, and for fractures of both bones of the forearm and fractures around the elbow. Fixation plates and screws are usually made of stainless steel. Other alloys, particularly titanium metals, are also frequently used.

In the ER, wounds after fracture fixation should be treated like all other wounds and inspected for redness, erythema, and swelling suggestive of infection. Avoid squeezing wounds, as pus can be forced deeper into the wound. Increased pain after plating can also indicate loosening. Decrease activity in the involved extremity and send the patient to the treating physician so that current x-rays can be compared to previous ones.

As swelling decreases after surgery on an open fracture, two conditions may occur that trouble patients. The first is the appearance of the ecchymosis in the dependent part of the

FIGURE 11-1 Open reduction and internal fixation of midshaft fractures of both forearm bones.

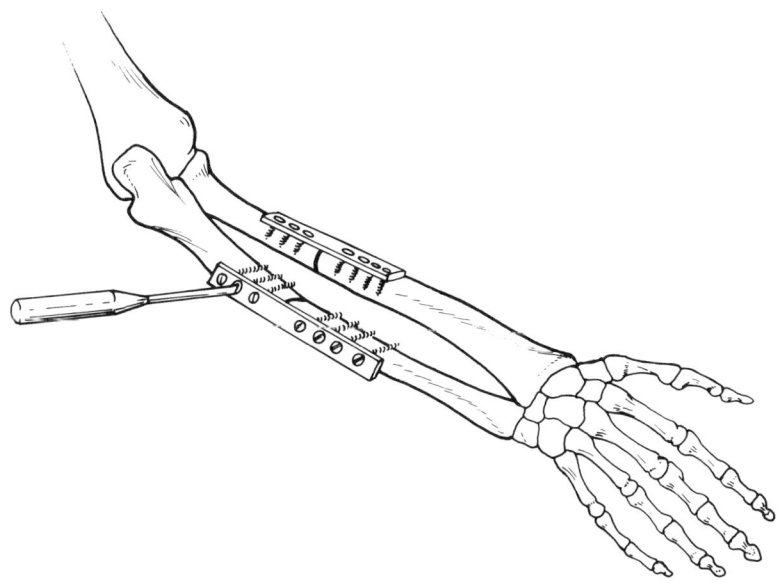

limb. For example, after fixation of a fibula fracture, the heel often first turns blue and then surrounding areas become yellow as blood becomes dependent and is gradually absorbed. Patients are worried about this and often seek medical advice. Second, there may be swelling just after an operation, which slowly resolves. As this happens, the edges of plates, ends of wires, and heads of screws become prominent and palpable. Patients find this alarming and often need reassurance. It is usually a simple matter to take out the appliance as a day surgery procedure after the fracture is solidly healed.

External fixateurs are perhaps the oldest form of bone instrumentation for fractures. These devices consist of screws, wires, or pins affixed to bone, which are then connected to clamps or rings to form a temporary exoskeleton. (See Figure 11-2.) The reduction of the fracture can be achieved either fluoroscopically or by direct visualization. The most common locations for external fixateurs are on the distal radius, the tibia, and the pelvis. Fixateur pins that go in on one side of the bone are called **half pins**. If they pass all the way through the bone and out the other side, they are called **transfixing pins.** Thin wires (Kirschner or K-wires) can also be used for transfixion.

The greatest problem with external fixation is caused by the pin tracts. Since the pin passes through the skin and into the bone, it serves as a conduit for bacteria. Pins may have some drainage. The percentage of pins that drain increases with the length of time the fixateur is in place. Loose pins also have drainage. The problem is to distinguish between the small amount of usually clear drainage that is present around many external fixateur pins and the drainage of an inflamed loose pin, which represents a potentially serious infection. Cultures of the drainage are really not helpful. Draining pins should be kept clean. Dry 4 × 4 gauzes can be used. Crusts can be removed with a little half-strength peroxide on a Q-tip. As swelling decreases, the skin may tent over the pins as it emerges from bone. Here local anesthesia and a small incision may be necessary so the skin lies flat around the pin. This tenting makes pin care more difficult and painful. Hoffmann, the

FIGURE 11-2 External fixateur.

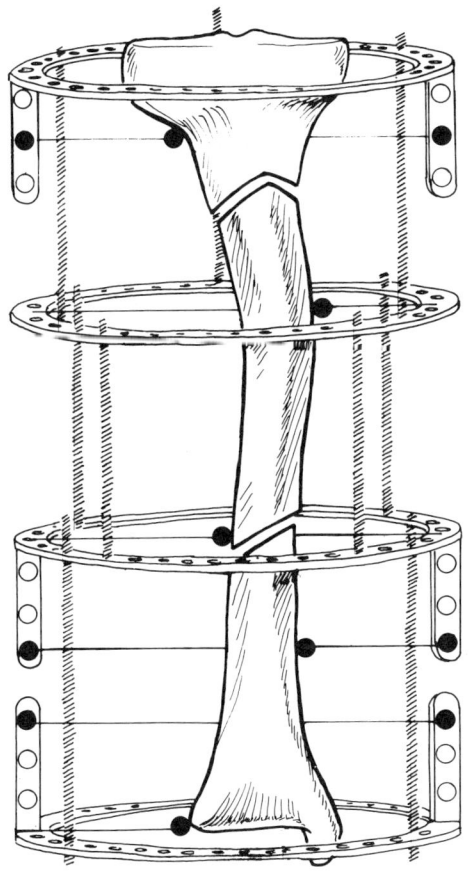

designer of the most commonly used external fixateur, once said the three commandments of external fixation are "release the skin, release the skin, release the skin!"

When patients who have had fracture fixation appear in the ER, the most difficult question is what to do about pain. Treatment with dispatch is the first thing that will help; the longer they wait in the ER, the more they will hurt. Second, be certain they have follow-up with a specialist in a few days. Third, understand that these conditions really do hurt and the pain is usually relieved only with narcotic pain medication. In addition, the patient must be taught that decreased activity and elevation of the limb helps greatly.

Pain after orthopedic injury lasts much longer than pain after abdominal surgery. Bone healing takes months. It is sensible to instruct the patient in elevation and decreased activity, arrange for prompt follow-up, and provide for an appropriate, small amount of narcotic pain medicine. Write prescriptions carefully. If the patient is to be seen tomorrow and you prescribe four tablets with an instruction to take one every six hours as needed for pain, spell out <u>four</u> so that the numeral *4* cannot be altered to *40*. The trouble times for patients are particularly in the evening, when they have difficulty falling asleep. Very often myoclonic jerks, which are part of the normal process of falling asleep, cause alarming involuntary movement of an injured extremity. The patient's first few trials of limb dependency in a recently treated fracture can be intensely unpleasant, as are the first few motions of a repaired joint. Understand these problems and give an adequate prescription for pain medicine.

Chapter 12
Traction and Suspension

In the traditional picture, the orthopedic patient, covered in bandages, lies in bed with an overhead frame, both arms and legs hanging by ropes and pulleys. Traction and suspension have been integral parts of the treatment of long-bone injuries since antiquity. Only in recent years have these methods ceased to be the mainstay of the care of long-bone fractures and been limited mostly to the preoperative period.

Some definitions are in order. **Suspension** is the use of frames and weights to elevate an extremity off the bed. In **traction** a force is applied to lengthen or extend a limb. This force acts over time to reduce a deformity and restore the normal configuration of the extremity.

Simple straight-out traction through a pulley will reduce the painful muscle forces that maintain fracture displacement, e.g., a femoral shaft fracture. In arranging traction in a severely ill, unconscious patient, it is critical to make certain that pressure points do not develop. In particular, the heel should be well protected. A heel sore or pressure point that develops during the early care of the patient can lead to skin breakdown or nerve palsy, which can become a greater problem than the initial injury.

Traction can be applied either to the skin or to the bony skeleton. The term **skin traction** is used when a soft dressing is bound to the limb and a traction apparatus is attached to the soft dressing. So-called "Buck's traction," in which a prefabricated, disposable foam boot is placed on the leg, is an example of skin traction. The "Buck's boot" is placed on clean, dry skin and is held by Velcro fasteners.

Skin traction is a convenient method used most commonly in children and the elderly who have injuries where powerful muscles are not creating deformity. It is appropriate for an elderly patient who has suffered a femoral neck fracture. This traction is made in a straight line with the leg, and a single pulley is placed at the end of the bed. Only three to five pounds of traction should be used. In the elderly patient with a femoral neck fracture, the patient should be placed in Buck's traction in the emergency room. Sandbags should be placed around the thigh to control rotation and make the patient more comfortable. Proper positioning in traction also reduces the amount of perioperative bleeding.

For skeletal traction, transfixing pins are inserted through the bony skeleton, such as in the distal femur or proximal tibia; the traction apparatus is then applied to the pin. The most common locations for skeletal traction are the proximal tibia, followed by the distal femur, the calcaneus, the olecranon, and the metacarpals. The advantage of skeletal traction over skin traction is that heavier weights can be applied to the limb to reduce deformity. In general, 15–20 lb (7.5–10 kg) of traction are placed on a pin through the distal femur, and 10-15 lb on a pin in the proximal tibia. With skin traction only 3–5 lb of continuous traction can be applied. Skeletal traction is an invasive procedure and carries with it the risks of pin-tract infection and damage to neurovascular structures if placed incorrectly. However, with proper placement and aseptic technique these risks are significantly reduced. The use of skeletal traction has associated with it a very low complication rate, probably because it is used only for a short period until a definitive procedure can be performed. A skeletal traction pin can be placed in the emergency room into the proximal tibia, for example, by prepping the skin as a sterile field, injecting local anesthetic in the skin and onto the periosteum, and inserting the pin dorsal and inferior to the tibial tubercle with a hand brace.

Nontransfixing traction is most commonly used for skull traction. In cases of cervical spine injuries, for example, Gardner-Wells tongs are attached to the patient's skull and, with the patient in the supine position, the traction apparatus is attached to the tongs.

Limbs are often suspended to reduce swelling and/or control bleeding. This is an especially useful technique for forearm and hand injuries, where the use of a canvas arm sling or foam block to suspend the injured upper extremity over the level of the heart reduces swelling and controls bleeding.

Many of the classic forms of lower limb traction are actually combinations of traction and suspension, where a metal frame called a **Thomas splint** is often used with a knee attachment called a **Pearson attachment** to suspend the lower extremity (Figure 12-1). This puts the hip and knee in a flexed position, so the leg is parallel to the bed. Traction is made through a Steinmann pin that has been placed in the proximal tibia. The thick-threaded Steinmann pins are in contrast to smoother Kirschner wires (K-wires), which are tensioned with a wire tensioning bow. Tensioning of the wire makes it stiffer, so it does not bend when weights are placed on it. Traction suspension systems based on either Steinmann pins or K-wires are in common orthopedic practice (Table 12-1).

TABLE 12-1 Kit for Skeletal Traction

Skin prep solution

1% lidocaine

Syringe, needles

Knife blade and handle

Sterile drapes

Gloves

Traction pins

Traction bows

Hand brace and chuck

Pin caps

Sponges

Sharps disposable container

FIGURE 12-1 Thomas ring splint with Pearson attachment.

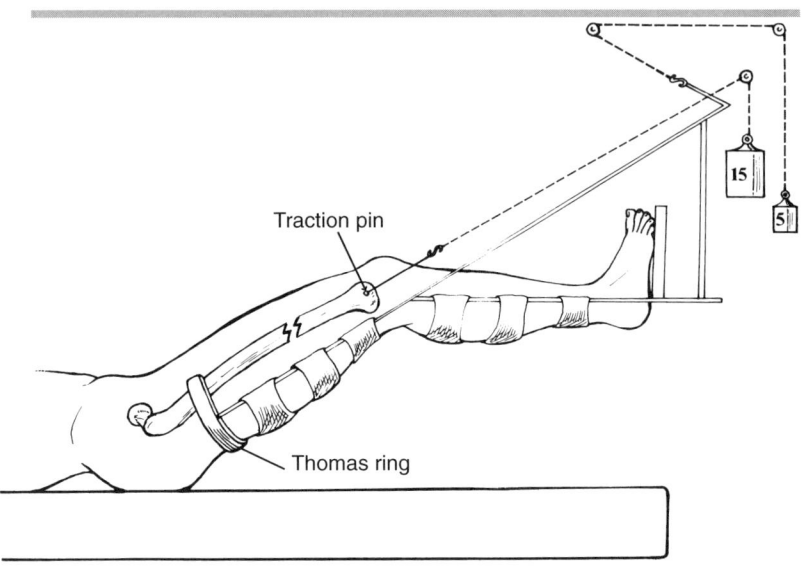

Chapter 13

Legal and Economic Aspects of Musculoskeletal Injury

Musculoskeletal injury is a leading cause of disability. Unlike other major processes affecting productivity—e.g., cancer or myocardial infarction—musculoskeletal conditions can, for the most part, be treated with excellent recovery. For injuries, however, the process draws in the legal profession, because recovery is assigned an economic value that includes the cost of the treatment, the extent of permanent incapacity, and lost wages. In the negotiation responsibility is determined and a dollar value assessed.

The essence of the system is that a happening (the accident) puts into play a sequence of events that causes economic damage and for which restitution is possible. If I hit your car and damage a fender, I owe you the value of the repair or replacement. It is critical to remember that the civil system of law is not intended to punish wrongdoing or reward injured pride, but to provide restoration for economic damages.

The cause-effect, repayment equation has a deadly logic of its own. Volkswagen or vintage Jaguar—the value lost is the value to be replaced. If you, however, were driving the Jaguar the wrong way down a one-way street, you may share in the responsibility for the event—contributory negligence. In this case, the amount of damage to be repaid is not changed, only its apportionment. The rules vary from jurisdiction to jurisdiction.

The written record of the first medical encounter has monstrous importance in sifting through the consequences of an accident. For example, if a patient is not wearing a seat belt and is thrown from a vehicle, the failure to "buckle up" may be contributory negligence. If the seat belt fails, perhaps its manufacturer is partially liable. These facts, though of little importance to the treating physician, are the crucial bits of evidence to be debated by the involved parties, each represented by a lawyer, whose pay is often determined by how much of the damages the lawyer can avoid having the client pay.

To settle a claim a lawsuit may be filed. The involved parties then have a right to *discover* what the facts are. Most disputes are settled before they ever reach trial in this "discovery" phase. The venue for discovery is a deposition. Lawyers have the right to command your appearance at a deposition. Failure to cooperate can lead to a contempt citation and imprisonment. Practically, depositions are scheduled to suit your convenience. Since everyone is reasonably paid for their time, the deponent physician—unless defending against a malpractice suit—should also expect reasonable hourly compensation.

The law, justice, and the truth do not always coincide. The words a lawyer may require to unlock the treasure chest are shaped by judicial opinions in the jurisdiction where the matter is brought. Each municipality, each state, and every level of the federal system has its own rules. The nature of the matter under dispute and the skill of the firm filing the case determine where it will be heard and how the game will be played.

The proximate cause of a chain of events that results in damages that can be compensated may be described differently by honest observers of the event. Ultimately, the jurors who review the case will arrive at a decision. As physicians, we view the differential diagnosis as a continuum in which each possibility can be assigned a probability value. In medical testimony a different standard is usually applied. One must determine whether an event is "more likely than not." If it is, the opinion is based in "reasonable medical probability." For example, in my opinion, based in reasonable medical probability, the patient broke her leg in the car accident. Implicit, however, is the concept that anything is possible.

Malpractice is the unpleasant accusation that a failure of performance by a physician is the cause of damages. This failure is measured against "the standard of care," which is what most prudent physicians would do in similar circumstances.

Often failures do not result in damages, and without recoverable damages there can never be a malpractice case. On the other hand, large damages associated with complications often are the motivating factors for lawyers. Loss of a limb is a good example. This type of problem in a previously healthy, employed patient may result in great economic damage. Since legal fees are computed as a percentage of the final reward, the greater the damage the greater the interest. An accusation of malpractice may be one of the factors considered in trying to determine the proximate cause of a costly outcome.

The physician who writes plainly, listens to each question attentively, answers thoughtfully and succinctly and appraises medical-legal problems honestly and without criticism of lawyers and/or 'the system' will do well for the profession and his/her patients.

PART II
REGIONAL INJURIES

Chapter 14

Fractures and Dislocations about the Shoulder

Trauma about the shoulder is terrifically painful. However, as an isolated injury from a fall or from sports, these conditions are rarely permanently disabling.

The first step in evaluating the shoulder is inspection. The common injuries—clavicle fracture, acromioclavicular separation (Figure 14-1), shoulder dislocation, and surgical neck fracture—can often be diagnosed by inspection. Because of the proximity of the brachial plexus to the shoulder constellation, injuries that involve the shoulder require full evaluation of the brachial plexus (Figure 14-2) to ensure that it is grossly intact. This can be done by having the patient make a fist, extend the thumb, and "make a muscle" with the biceps. Patients with neurologic dysfunction need to be admitted. The next step is to palpate along the clavicle, acromion, coracoid, scapula, and humerus to detect tenderness, crepitus, or gross deformity that was not revealed during inspection. Passive range of motion should be performed to determine if there is limitation. Cold packs are helpful in relieving pain while radiographs are taken.

In injuries involving the shoulder, one should get an AP and one other view. The AP x-ray is often taken perpendicular to the coronal plane.

FIGURE 14-1 Severe (grade III) acromioclavicular separation in a football player. Note that the end of the clavicle does not line up with the acromion, and the distance between the coracoid and the clavicle is increased.

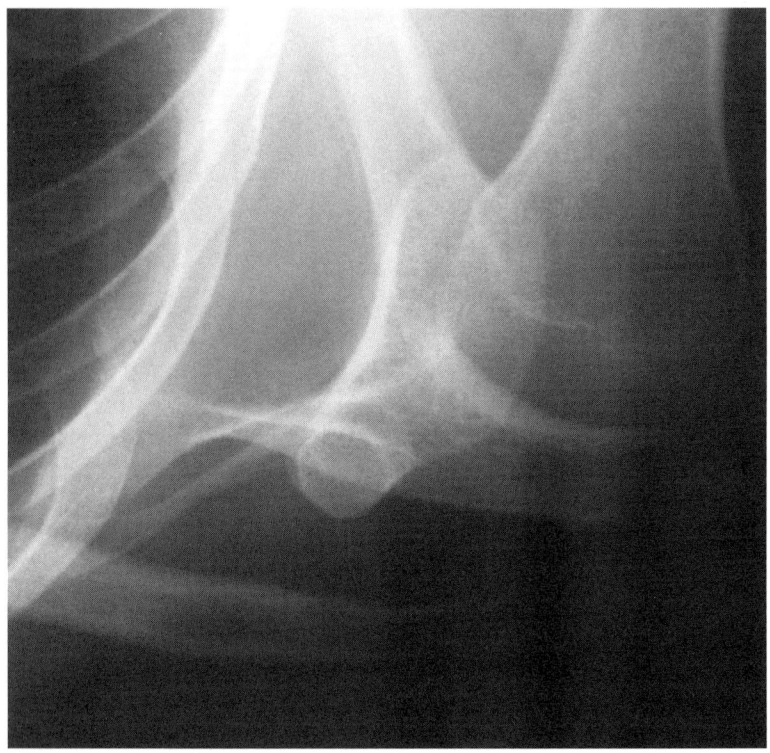

FIGURE 14-2 The shoulder constellation. In examining the shoulder on x-ray, one should look for: (1) acromioclavicular separation—the normal relationship between the acromion and clavicle should be coplanar, (2) fractures of the greater tuberosity, the surgical neck of the humerus, and the clavicle, and (3) dislocation of the humeral head. The most common type of dislocation is anterior; the one most often missed is posterior.

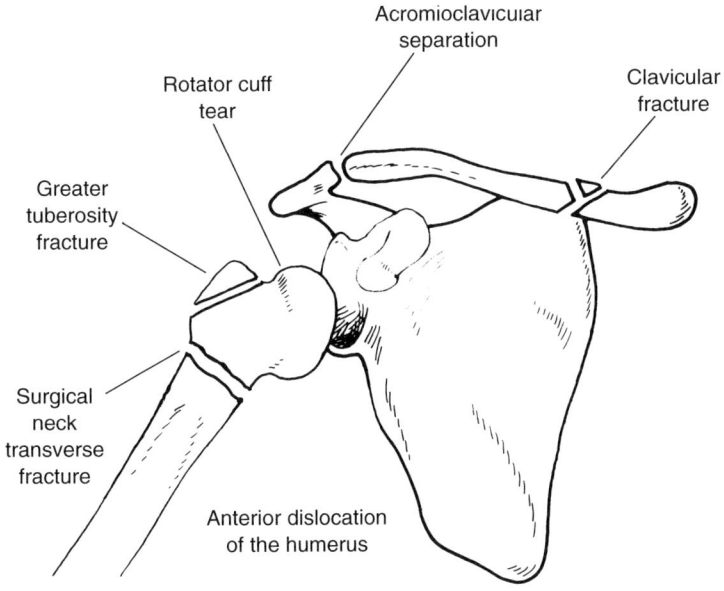

PROXIMAL HUMERUS FRACTURES

Fractures of the proximal humerus are common injuries. The two most common proximal humerus fractures are avulsion of the greater tuberosity with the insertion of the rotation cuff and fracture below the head and tuberosities of the humerus at the surgical neck. As long as anatomic relationships are approximately correct and the shaft of the humerus is reasonably aligned with the head, the treatment of these fractures is an arm sling, pain medication, local ice for pain control and prompt followup. Children who fall from a height, young adults in motor cycle accidents and elderly patients in auto collisions infrequently sustain complex fractures which displace the humerus shaft from the head or shatter the articular surface. These are complex problems which require multiple special x rays, C.T. scans and/or fluoroscopic evaluation. An x ray in a second plate such as a transthoracic, or scapular *Y*-x ray can be helpful in assessing the pathology. Either percutaneous pinning or open reduction and plate fixation may be necessary. These operations are performed subacutely, and if is appropriate to arrange for care of the patient with an isolated injury on an outpatient basis. With marked joint surface comminution, an endoprosthetic replacement may be performed.

CLAVICLE FRACTURES

More than three-fourths of all clavicle fractures involve the middle third of the clavicle, the majority being treated nonsurgically with a figure-of-eight soft clavicle straps. Surgery is indicated if there is associated neurovascular compromise marked displacement with tenting of the skin by the fractured bone ending or open fractures. The surgical treatment of choice is ORIF with or without bone graft.

SCAPULA FRACTURES

To fracture the scapula, high energy is usually involved. The majority of these fractures are treated nonsurgically with a sling. This is because the scapula is surrounded by highly vascular musculature, which aids in the rapid healing of the fracture site. Fractures that require surgery involve fractures through the glenoid, which can lead to either instability or arthrosis.

SHOULDER DISLOCATIONS

The most common of all dislocations are those of the shoulder. Anterior dislocation is most frequent and occurs secondary to external rotation of an abducted arm. The patient presents with loss of normal fullness of the front of the shoulder and with pain. The neurovascular bundle passes anterior to the glenohumeral joint. Thus, injury to the axillary nerve as well as the median, ulna, and radial nerves need to be evaluated.

A dislocated shoulder is reduced by axial traction (sometimes analgesia and muscle relaxation are needed) and may be facilitated by placing the patient prone. First-time dislocators need a sling with a strap or swathe to keep the arm in internal rotation (against the body). If the shoulder has been "out" for more than a few hours or if there is an associated humeral head fracture or avulsion of the greater tuberosity, as is common in the elderly population, a specialty consult is appropriate. For patients with recurrent dislocations surgery should be considered. However, the shoulder is reduced in the emergency room, and repair is arranged as an elective procedure. In instances where closed reduction is unsuccessful, particularly where the shoulder has been dislocated for hours, the specialist will probably arrange for reduction under anesthesia. Rarely, an open reduction and repair will be necessary on an acute basis.

Anterior dislocations of the shoulder are most common, but *posterior dislocations* are most often missed. The patient will present with the arm in adduction and internal rotation and will be unable to abduct or externally rotate the arm. On exam, there is a protruding mass in the posterior aspect of the shoulder. Again, axial traction is applied with appropriate force to reposition the humeral head anteriorly.

Rotator cuff injuries are usually secondary to overuse or trauma via an inflammatory process. The patient will have rotator cuff muscular tenderness and have a history of pain with forward flexion, abduction, and external rotation. The order of insertion of the external rotators on the humerus from posterior to anterior can be remembered by the mnemonic **SITS** (supraspinatus, infraspinatus, teres minor, and subscapularis). On x-ray, one will see elevation of the humeral head on the glenoid fossa with complete rotator cuff rupture. This is not always the case, and further radiographic evaluation is performed with first an ultrasound and then an arthrogram and then MRI (if necessary).

Other painful musculoskeletal conditions, including bicipital tendinitis and cervical radiculopathy, can present as shoulder pain. The lack of a definite injury and presence of pain on palpation over the affected tendons or over the cervical spinous processes are helpful findings for making these diagnoses.

Table 14-1 outlines pathology and cause of musculoskeletal shoulder problems.

TABLE 14-1 Fractures and Dislocations about the Shoulder

PATHOLOGY	SYMPTOM/CAUSE
Clavicle fracture	Swollen, sore, with crepitus at the fracture
Acromioclavicular separation	Point tenderness at the AC joint
Rotator cuff tear	Middle-aged patient with decreased power of abduction and external rotation
Anterior dislocation of humerus	Normal fullness gone, pain
Surgical neck fracture	Old age, deformity

Chapter 15
Fractures of the Humerus Shaft

The humerus is fractured less commonly than the femur or the tibia. The diagnosis is easy to make clinically. Pain and deformity are evident. On the x-ray the fracture pattern is more important than the amount of displacement or angulation. How bent or how far apart the fractured bone ends lie depends on how the arm is positioned on the x-ray plate when the film is taken. It takes skill to get two x-rays in different planes without hurting the patient. Often a cross chest view helps. Fractures are described by location (upper, middle, lower third), geometry (transverse, oblique, spiral), and amount of comminution (see Chapter 22). Remember to get x-rays of the shoulder and elbow to find associated fractures in the same arm.

Begin the evaluation by examining for and recording radial nerve function (Figure 15-1). Spiral fractures of the humerus are associated with *radial nerve* injury, because the course of the nerve lies in close proximity to the humerus at the junction of the middle and distal thirds of the humerus. Therefore, begin your evaluation by examining for radial nerve function. If nerve function is diminished after reduction and splinting, the nerve may need to be surgically explored and released. Patients with radial nerve palsy and humerus shaft fracture are carefully observed and often treated with exploration of the nerve and fracture fixation with a bone plate or an intramedullary nail. Other indications for early operation include the presence of soft tissue interposed between fracture fragments and vascular

FIGURE 15-1 Accident—the Painful Arm. In the event of a painful deformed arm, it is imperative to ascertain whether there is neurovascular compromise by assessing the patient's pulses and nerve function. If the patient is neurovascularly intact, splint the arm and have the patient return for follow-up in 2 to 5 days for definitive fracture management.

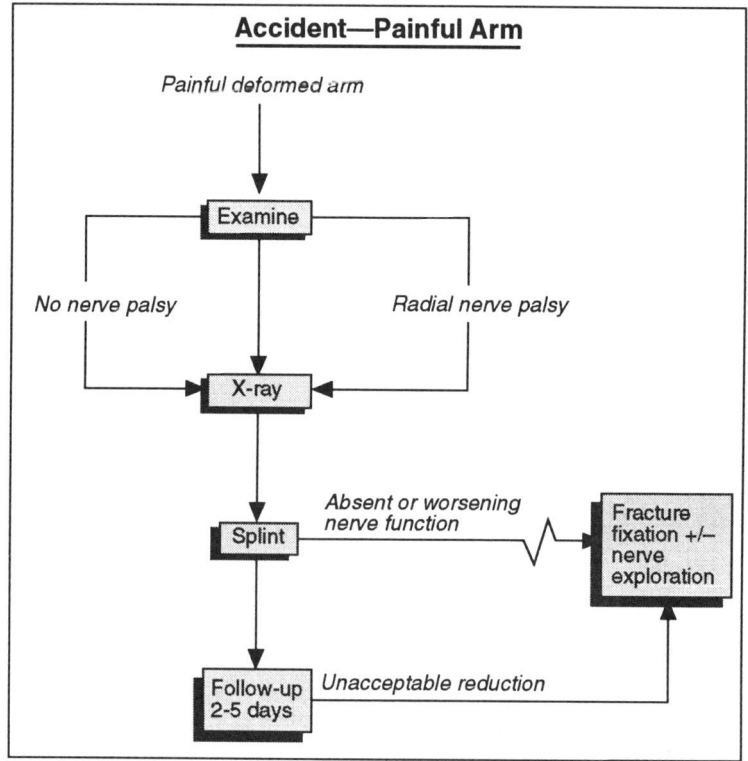

compromise. Combined injuries or unstable fractures may be operated on so that the patient gains use of the arm while the fracture is healing. Choice of method depends on the problem and the surgeon's training and judgment.

Healing in a significant percentage of displaced fractures of the humerus is delayed. When this occurs, securing union can be a real challenge. The disability from loss of use of the dominant upper limb can be severe.

In general, when a long-bone fracture such as a humerus fracture takes more than six months to heal, it is spoken of as a **delayed union.** If healing has not taken place at the end of a year's treatment, then a **nonunion** or **pseudoarthrosis** is present.

The radial nerve innervates the wrist extensors. Ask the patient to dorsiflex the wrist or to extend (hitchhike) the thumb. Treatment of humerus shaft fractures is usually nonoperative with splints or braces. Precise bone alignment is not critical. Shortening, rotation, or angulation do not cause the same functional problem in the upper limb as they do in the lower one (Figures 15-2A, B, C).

Initial splinting to reduce motion between fracture fragments prevents nerve damage, increases patient comfort, and may prevent disturbances of fracture healing. The application of a comfortable upper arm splint or the adjustment of a long arm cast to maintain fracture reduction requires considerable skill.

A special cast is sometimes used that extends from the hand just above the elbow. The position of the fracture can be adjusted by placing loops on the cast and suspending the cast from the neck. This "hanging arm cast" may be used initially but has the risk of distracting the fracture and delaying union.

The minimally stable displaced fracture can usually be treated nonoperatively in the ER and sent home. A coaptation splint (also known as sandwich splint) is applied to the humerus. This splint is made by taking plaster material with cast padding on both sides and extending it from the acromion down around the elbow, then proximal to the axilla. It is held in place with a loose bandage (*Note:* Keep the elbow at 90°). A sling can then be used to support the arm.

FIGURE 15-2 *A.* A bending fracture of the humerus shaft in an 18-year-old woman with multiple injuries. Emergent treatment was a splint.

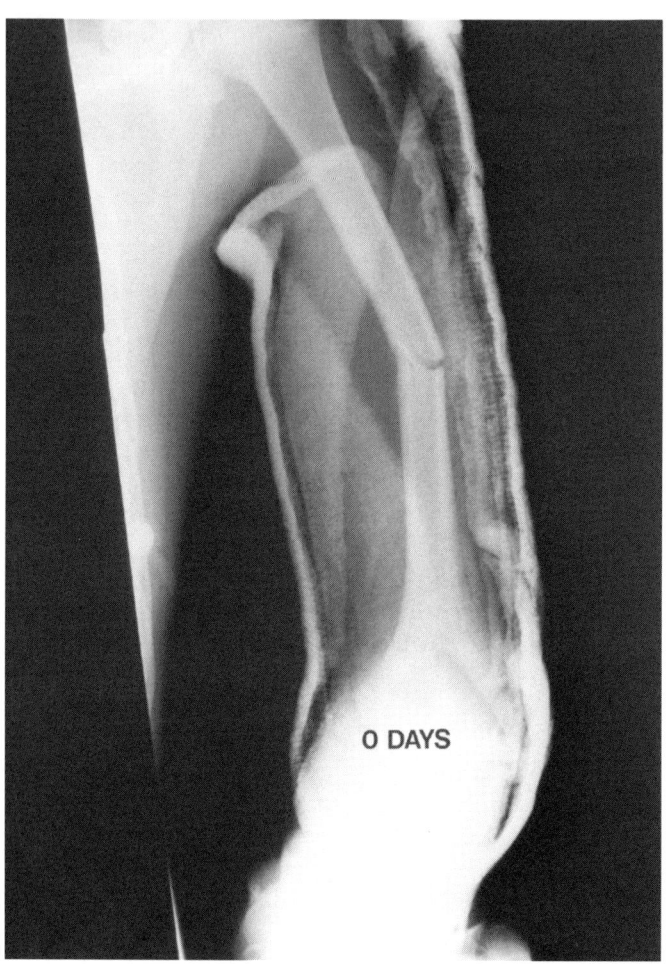

FRACTURES OF THE HUMERUS SHAFT

FIGURE 15-2 *(Continued) B.* At the time of fixation of her fracture, an external fixateur was placed on the humerus.

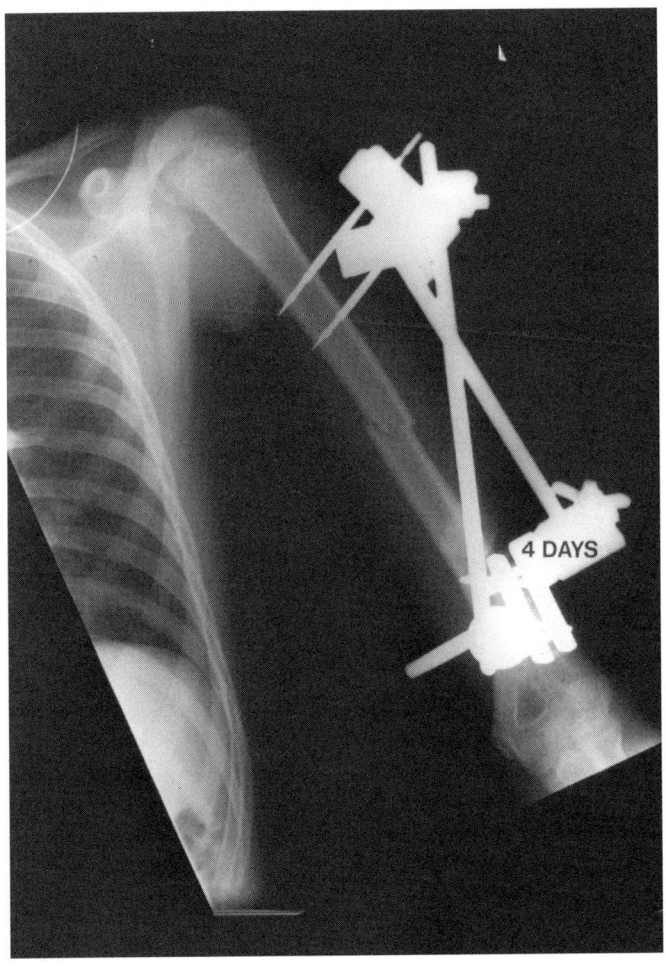

FIGURE 15-2 *(Continued)* **C. The fracture healed well.**

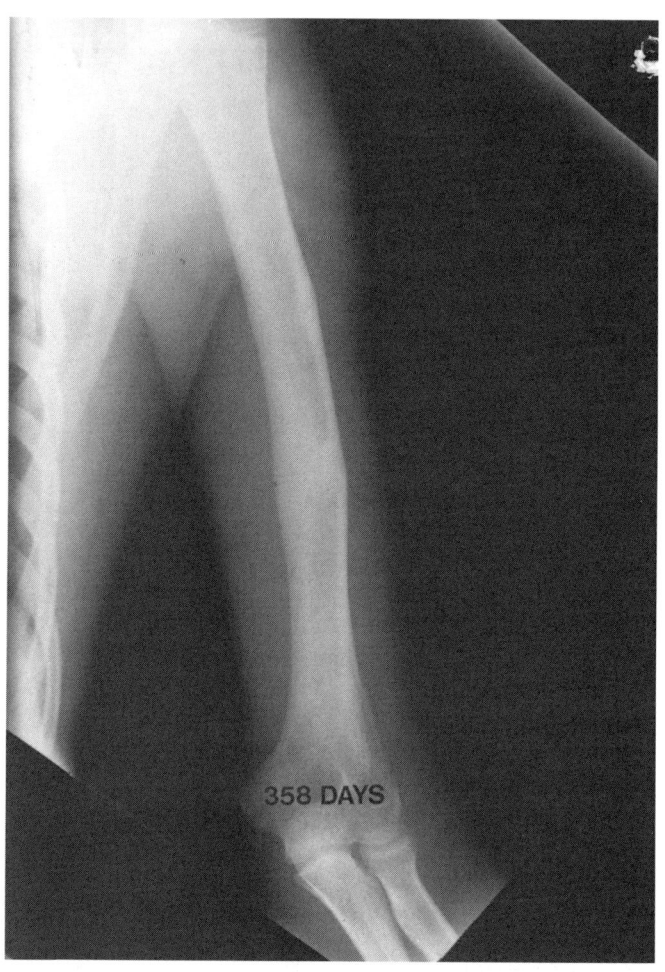

At the end of splinting, postreduction x-rays are taken. It is important to learn how to look at radiographs with the patient. Lay persons are fascinated by the concrete representation of injury. They may ask questions. Learn to listen and answer—you will learn a lot. What is clear to you may not be what they are thinking about. They may point, for example, to the coracoid process and ask if that is the fracture. When there is some displacement of fragments, which is allowable for good functional healing, they may be fearful and concerned. Discuss the displacement and provide the facts. A broken bone is not any more normal than a broken plate. After all, as one eminent orthopedist tells his patients: You broke God's bone!

Chapter 16
Elbow Injuries

The elbow joint allows rotation of the forearm (pronation-supination) through a range of flexion-extension by combining a rotating ball-to-disk articulation (capitulum to radial head) with a hinge joint (trochlea to olecranon). This complex mechanism can be contused, fractured, or dislocated. You can remember what articulates with what with the mnemonic **CRiTOe** (**C**apitellum, **R**adial head, **i**nternal epicondyle, **T**rochlea, **O**lecranon, **e**xternal epicondyle).

Elbow pain can also occur because of repetitive use. Characteristic locations are the epiphysis of the capitellum (**Little League elbow**), the external epicondyle (**tennis elbow**), and the tip of the olecranon (**stockbroker's elbow**).

In adults, gross displacement from fracture or dislocation of the elbow requires careful evaluation of the neurovascular status and prompt treatment. Commonly, however, patients sustain a jammed elbow from a fall on the outstretched hand or direct trauma to the olecranon. The subtle x-ray findings following minimal trauma are easy to overlook. Fortunately, patients with a painful elbow and possible minor impactions of the radial head, fractures of the coronoid process, and other associated cracks are safely treated in a sling.

For these minor injuries place the elbow at a right angle (90° to the floor), and wrap from the palm to the arm with cast padding, and apply an ACE bandage loosely. Place the arm in a simple cradle arm sling and arrange for follow-up in a few days.

A dislocated elbow can be reduced by axial traction on the forearm and direct pressure on the tip of the olecranon. With good, steady traction, keeping the elbow in the position one finds it, slowly flex and push the tip of the olecranon around the trochlea. If an elbow cannot easily be reduced, an anesthetic is needed. Be sure to distinguish between straightforward dislocations and dislocations associated with fractures. Fracture dislocations can be made more complex by nonoperative manipulation. A common association is a fracture of the proximal ulna with dislocated radial head—**Monteggia's fracture**. Patients with displaced supracondylar fractures, or displaced fractures of the capitellum, trochlea, olecranon, or radial head, are hospitalized (Figure 16-1). These injuries will usually require open reduction and internal fixation.

While precision in diagnosis of minor injuries to the adult elbow is important, interpretation of the initial x-ray in children's elbow injuries is important and difficult. In children, not only can the diagnosis be difficult, but also treatment is hazardous, because posttraumatic swelling can cause permanent contracture (**Volkmann's ischemic contracture**). The diagnosis of injury from plain x-rays is difficult because the pediatric elbow consists mostly of cartilage. Broken cartilage does not show a fracture line on x-ray. The presence of a fracture is deduced by the relative positions of the epiphyseal growth centers. Mentally fill in the outline of the cartilage block and you will see the fracture clearly.

Therefore, in patients under 10 years of age, an x-ray of the opposite elbow positioned like the injured elbow is helpful (Figure 16-2). The mnemonic for the order of appearance of the epiphyses is **CRITOE,** as defined at the beginning of this chapter. When the comparison x-ray and injured elbow film are taken in the same position, the epiphyses lie in similar locations. Displacement of an epiphysis or obvious fracture is a specialty problem. A child will not move an injured joint. If there is local pain in the elbow, and elevation of the articular fat pad (a sign of effusion), a sling and follow-up in a few days are indicated. Dislocation of the radial head occurs when a worried parent pulls a toddler away from danger. The characteristic presentation is pain and inability to turn the forearm. Reduction often occurs when the x-ray technician supinates the forearm for an x-ray.

FIGURE 16-1   A displaced fracture of the lateral (trochlea) condyle and epicondyle of the distal humerus. The joint is not congruent. This fracture will require open reduction. It is prudent to splint the arm and admit the patient preoperatively, since this injury carries a risk of compartment syndrome.

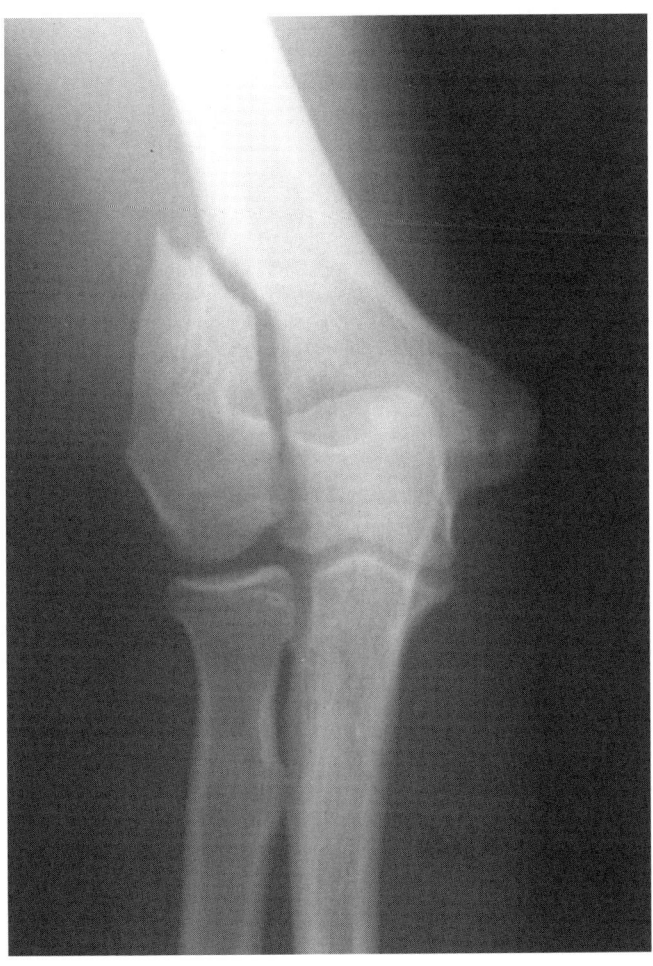

FIGURE 16-2   The elbow x-ray. In the event of a painful elbow, obtain an elbow x-ray (AP and lateral). Examine the film for a fat pad sign, which indicates an effusion. If present, you must rule out a fracture. Draw a line down the anterior border of the humerus. It should pass through the anterior one-third to one-half of the capitellum. If it intersects one-third, a supracondylar fracture should be suspected. A line drawn down the radius should transect the capitulum. If it does not, a radial head dislocation should be suspected.

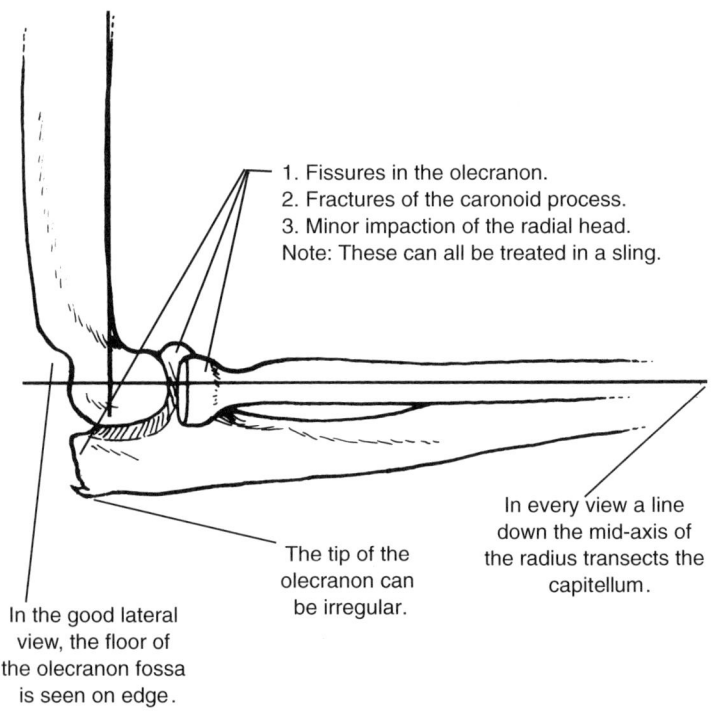

Always recheck the pulse after splinting an elbow fracture in a child. If the pulse is initially absent, the problem is an orthopedic emergency (see Chapter 6). If the pulse is diminished after splinting, the splints should be removed and the arm repositioned. A case that has shown evidence of vascular compromise needs careful inpatient observation, even though a dramatically displaced fracture has been reduced.

Another word about x-rays is appropriate. Radiographs are indispensable, not only for the evaluation of trauma but also for follow-up. X-ray films are cumbersome, damaged by water, difficult to reproduce with good detail, and incredibly easy to misplace. Patients, doctors, and the mail are all unreliable in delivering them to the next place they are needed to aid the physician in the treatment of the patient. Thoughtful traumatologists attempt at least to get them read, filed appropriately, and available for follow-up care. Films can generally be signed out of a radiology department and brought to the physician's office on the day of reexamination. This discussion is pertinent to elbow x-rays, as well as hand, foot, and cervical spine films. Often additional findings are discovered by the radiologist who has a chance to review the films in a quiet setting at a reasonable time of day. An occult missed fracture of the radial head, for example, is best dealt with by calling the office of the physician to whom the patient was referred. The initial treatment (bulky dressing, sling) is not really changed because of the radiographic findings, and bringing the patient back to the emergency room on an urgent basis is not productive. Surely x-ray films, relics of the nineteenth century, will be replaced by electronic images before too long.

Chapter 17

Forearm Fractures

The forearm is a two-bone unit comprised of the ulna and radius. Generally, when one bone is fractured and displaced, the other is also fractured or dislocated. Two Italians described this principle: a fracture of the proximal ulna with dislocation of the radial head is called **Monteggia's fracture,** and fracture of the distal radius with dislocation of the distal ulna is **Galeazzi's fracture.** The exception to this general principle is an isolated fracture of the ulna caused by a direct blow—when the arm is held up to parry away the blow from a truncheon. The result is termed a **night-stick** or **parry fracture.** This night-stick fracture can be splinted and sent for follow-up, while both bone fractures and fracture dislocations require manipulation and, in adults, operative fixation.

Inspect the forearm for open wounds and gross deformity. Assess circulation by checking the radial and ulnar pulses or by squeezing the fingertips and looking for capillary refill. Evaluate neurologic function by having the patient make a fist (median nerve), "hitchhike" the thumb (radial nerve), and bring out the little finger (ulnar nerve).

A complete x-ray examination of the forearm always includes films of the wrist and elbow joint. These views should be at right angles to each other, but the distortion of the fractured forearm can make definition of the projections difficult. The action of the muscles, particularly the pronator teres, which rotates the broken radius, displaces the fractured ends of the bone.

Children's fractures can usually be managed in the emergency department. Stable fractures are placed in a sandwich splint—one plaster slab anterior and one slab dorsal. Taking one long splint around the elbow so that it resembles a barbecue tong controls forearm rotation. Remember that the *pronator* controls the forearm. The prone, face-down, or palm-down hand deposits coins in the palm-up, *supine*, supinated hand of a panhandler. Fractures of the forearm proximal to the pronator insertion in the middle third of the radius are splinted in supination, fractures in the middle third of the radius in neutral, and distal third fractures in pronation.

Unstable fractures are reduced under systemic intravenous sedation or a regional anesthetic. The patient should be monitored with a pulse oximeter. If available, an image intensifier is the best way to control the reduction. In incomplete (**greenstick**) fractures of the radius or ulnar shaft, the fractures are completed so the bone will heal straight. As the bone is grasped and straightened there will be an audible "pop." Consider placing the child's parents where they cannot hear the noise. Use a long arm cast to maintain the reduction, but then be cautious of swelling. The closed cast can cause a compartment syndrome and death of muscle (**Volkmann's contracture**). This produces a dysfunctional claw hand. Either split the cast or admit the patient to observe for swelling—or better, do both.

In adults, fractures of the radial or ulnar shafts are initially treated with immobilization. Use a long arm, barbecue-tong splint or sandwich splints. The patient is generally hospitalized for definitive management with ORIF. Elevate the extremity and supply analgesics and ice packs. When both bones are fractured, plate fixation or possibly a combination with an intramedullary nail and or external fixateur will be used for treatment.

The "Italian fractures" of Monteggia and Galeazzi are best treated with plate fixation of the broken long bone. Often the dislocated joint is stable. However, in Monteggia's fracture the dislocated radial head must have torn the restraining annular ligament to have dislocated. The reduction is maintained by flexing the elbow to a right angle. Occasionally the head redislocates. Such patients will return to the emergency room and must, like patients with recurrent elbow dislocations, be reduced, resplinted, and have prompt follow-up arranged. Similarly, after treatment for Galeazzi's fracture the distal radioulnar joint (DRUJ) may be unstable. Grasp the distal radius in one hand and the distal ulnar in the other. Assess stability by moving the bones back and forth in relation to each other like a pair of maracas. After acute injury, the radius is plated, then the distal joint is assessed; if unstable, it can be pinned or repaired to control this problem.

Chapter 18

Wrist Injuries

Low-energy fractures of the distal radius (and ulna) and of the proximal carpal row (scaphoid, lunate, triquetrum) are the common consequences of simple falls on the hand. High-speed accidents produce shearing injuries to the distal radius and intercarpal fracture-dislocations, which can be complicated by median nerve compression.

In addition, there is a group of painful conditions often associated with repetitive use of the wrist and hand that frequently present as emergencies because they are intensely uncomfortable and interfere with work.

The common painful wrist conditions that may be caused by repetitive use are shown in Table 18-1. Patients with these conditions can all be placed in a wrist splint, given nonnarcotic, nonsteroidal, anti-inflammatory medication and referred to a specialist interested in hand conditions.

Fractures of the distal radius are common. Pain over the wrist or carpus after a fall on the outstretched hand with a negative x-ray is even more common. The triage of these injuries begins by recognizing the radiographic appearance of significant fractures and dislocations that require urgent reduction (Figure 18-1). On the PA view of the wrist the cartilage space around all the carpal bones and between the proximal carpal row and the radius is present and should be symmetric. On the lateral view the long-finger metacarpal, the capitate, the lunate, and the radius all lie on a line. If the relationships on x-ray are distorted, the patient will need consultation, reduction, and possible operative stabilization.

Examine the wrist for local tenderness to palpation in four key areas: over the distal radius, over the carpal scaphoid on the thumb (dorsal-lateral) side of the wrist, over the

TABLE 18-1 Painful Wrist Conditions Caused by Repetitive Use

CONDITION	SYMPTOMS	FINDINGS
Carpal tunnel syndrome	Numbness of pain in thumb, index, and long finger	Pain over the median nerve at the wrist accentuated by wrist flexion (**Phalen's test**)
DeQuervain's disease	Local swelling over thumb abductor tendons	Tenderness over abductors at the radial styloid accentuated by ulnar deviation (**Finkelstein's test**)
Peritendinitis calcarea	Burning pain over the wrist flexor or extensor insertions	Erythema suggesting infection Calcifications on x-ray
Keinboch-Preisler disease	Painful wrist motion and diminished strength	Cystic changes in scaphoid and/or lunate on x-ray
Carpo-metacarpal arthritis of the thumb	Pain at the base of the thumb	CMC arthritis of thumb on x-ray Grinding the base of the thumb metacarpal into the trapezium reproduces the pain

FIGURE 18-1 Accident—painful wrist. In the event of a painful wrist, one must first determine whether fracture or displacement has occurred. If neither has occurred, the wrist should be splinted and the patient sent home with pain medications. A patient with a Colles' fracture that is confirmed radiographically should undergo nonoperative reduction. If this is unsuccessful, it will be necessary to reduce the fracture operatively. If the fracture involves a carpal bone, the articular surface of the radius, or a nerve palsy, then operative reduction is necessary in order to restore normal architecture and function.

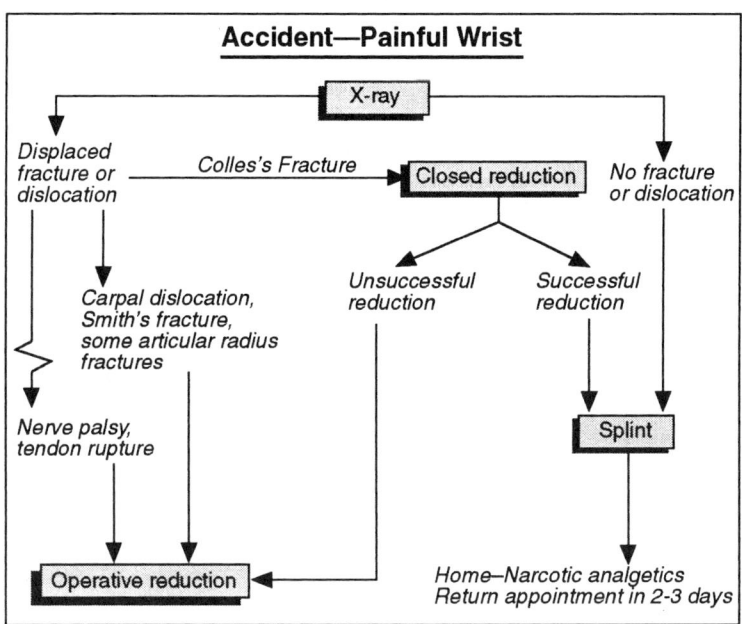

dorsum of the proximal carpal row, and over the ulnar styloid. Even if the x-ray appears negative, there may be damage to underlying structures (Figure 18-2). If there is pain to palpation over the scaphoid in the so-called "snuff box" formed by the thumb extensor tendons, a splint is always indicated. Since the carpal scaphoid (navicular) has a precarious blood supply, a splint including the thumb is applied for ten days to two weeks. If a nondisplaced fracture is evident on the follow-up x-ray, the patient can then be placed in a cast. The nondisplaced fracture line becomes visible because of bone resorption in the early phase of fracture healing. As a general principle, clinical evidence of fracture (local pain after injury) prompts treatment, even if the initial x-ray is normal.

The common distal radius fractures are lumped under the name **Colles'** fracture (Figure 18-3). The characteristic deformity is called a "dinner-fork" deformity because the wrist and hand look in profile like a fork turned tines down. This is because in most distal radius fractures, the wrist and hand are displaced dorsally and ulnarward. Reduction can be an emergency-room procedure. Under local infiltration or regional block anesthesia traction is applied to restore radial length, and direct pressure on the distal radius restores volar tilt. The arm is wrapped in cast padding, and palmar and dorsal plaster splints are placed. If the fracture is unstable and a circular cast is needed, it is advisable to place the patient in the hospital for observation or to split the cast and arrange for follow-up within 36 to 48 hours. Many unstable fractures and intra-articular fractures, particularly in adults, are better treated in external skeletal fixation. This can be accomplished by a specialist several days after the injury if the patient is splinted and sent promptly for follow-up treatment.

Many patients have disabling pain of the wrist after an injury to the hand without evidence of fracture or dislocation. These are important clinical problems, because torn ligaments can be intensely painful and cause disability. Included in this group of injuries are partial tears of the intercarpal ligaments, particularly the scapholunate ligaments, and damage to the distal radio-ulnar mechanism, the triangular fibrocartilage.

FIGURE 18-2 Lateral wrist x-ray. The mainstay of diagnosis with respect to wrist involvement is the radiograph. X-rays that should be obtained include PA, true lateral, and oblique. A lateral x-ray of the wrist in neutral position should have the third metacarpal, the capitate, the lunate, and the radius all lying on the same line. To help assess normal alignment, the scapholunate angle as depicted in the figure should be roughly 45°. On a PA view, three lines can be drawn: one on the proximal border of the scaphoid, lunate, and triquetrum bones; one on the distal border; and one on the proximal row of carpal bones. If any of these lines is broken, instability should be suspected.

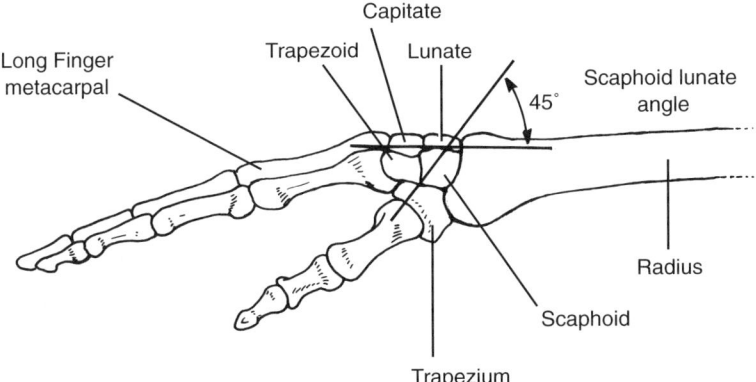

FIGURE 18-3 This nonarticular fracture of the distal radius in a seven year-old boy is the pediatric equivalent of Colles' fracture in the adult. Note excellent callus formation at eight weeks. Because of remodeling, the treatment of nonarticular children's fractures does not require operation or implants.

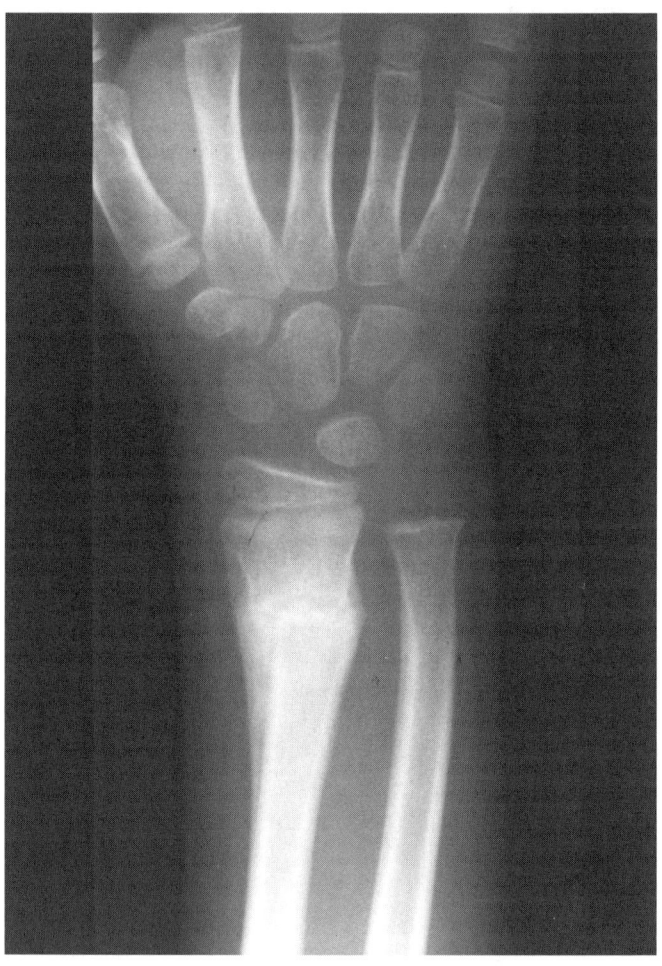

If these acute ligamentous tears are not immobilized with a splint, chronic instability with persistent painful clicking and loss of strength is more likely to be the result.

Intercarpal fractures and dislocations can be difficult to diagnose. The wrist may be massively swollen. The x-ray must be well centered. If you do not learn and remember the names of the carpal bones, it is hard to look at them individually and find the fractures. A mnemonic is helpful. If you don't like our silly one, use your own—beginning at the thumb:

Some	**S**caphoid
Lovers	**L**unate
Try	**T**riquetrum
Positions	**P**isiform
That	**T**rapezium
They	**T**rapezoid
Cannot	**C**apitate
Handle	**H**amate

The most common fracture of the carpus is a dorsal chip fracture of the triquetrum, seen as a fleck of bone dorsal to the proximal carpal row on the lateral x-ray. The fractured navicular is less common, but more significant. Dislocation patterns around the lunate are major massive injuries. Look at the carpal bones on x-ray until you know the normal pattern with confidence, and never hesitate to go over the films with a specialist until you are sure.

Chapter 19
Hand Fractures and Soft Tissue Injuries

We are incredibly dependent on our hands. We reach out to do so many things with them that our hands are at great risk of injury. They may be twisted, jammed, broken, crushed, burned, amputated, and hurt in any way imaginable. Today so much can be done to restore hands to their important functions that injured hands must be thoroughly evaluated and all injuries detected. Bleeding can be controlled by direct pressure. Deformity can be reduced. A numb finger will be forever numb unless the injury is appreciated and treatment planned.

Inspect the hand for any gross deformity, swelling, and ecchymosis. Next assess neurologic function by testing motor and sensory components of the median, radial, and ulnar nerves. Palpate the radial and ulnar arteries, assess capillary refill, and feel the digits to determine if they are pink and warm. Palpate the hand and each digit, noting any tenderness or crepitus. Measure the passive range of motion of each digit and assess the stability of each joint. On exam, ask the patient to flex digits 1–4; normally each digit should point to the tubercle of the scaphoid. If they do not, then a rotational deformity exists.

Just as the details of our lives are attended to by our own hands, so too does care of an injured hand require attention to detail. Draw a picture of a hand on the medical record. Mark the injuries. Sketch-in lacerations. Find out what the patient does with the hand and mark down handedness.

HAND FRACTURES

Hand fractures are common and are a significant source of disability. Unstable fractures and dislocation of phalanges and metacarpals are obvious clinically—the hand is deformed.

Distinguish on x-ray between diaphyseal fractures of the phalanges and metacarpals and articular fractures. The patterns of fractures can be described using the same language as for diaphyseal fractures of the long bones (see Chapter 22). Long spiral fractures of the metacarpals are common. Fractures of the proximal phalanges can run obliquely into the proximal interphalangeal joint. Note whether the fracture is intraarticular or wholly diaphyseal.

Anteroposterior, lateral, and oblique views of the hand should be obtained if a fracture is suspected. Examine each cortex for incongruity. Look closely at the proximal interphalangeal (PIP) joint and distal interphalangeal (DIP) joint for evidence of an intraarticular fracture, because often they involve disruption of the volar plate and or collateral ligaments, leading to dorsal displacement of the middle phalanx, and are considered unstable, requiring surgical intervention.

A deformed finger can usually be reduced by simply pulling the finger to straighten it. An intermetacarpal block can be administered by injecting 2–3 cc of 1% lidocaine into the web space between the metacarpal heads. Simple splinting, elevation, and pain medication are all appropriate, as is early follow-up with a hand specialist. If reduction is not easily accomplished, stop manipulation. There may be an unusual dislocation, involving entrapment of ligaments or tendons, that can only be reduced operatively. The most common dislocation with entrapment is when the head of the thumb metacarpal becomes entrapped. After reduction of a fracture or dislocation some of the injuries may be *unstable*—that is, deformity will recur in splints. A hand specialist needs to decide when operative treatment is required to maintain the reduced position. *Stable* fractures occur more frequently and present as a variety of fractures in tubular bones of the fingers and thumb. Foam-padded, malleable aluminum splints are used to hold these injured fingers. Alternatively, splint the injured finger to its uninjured adjacent finger (Buddy splinting). This also maintains correct alignment and allows some joint motion.

There are three common, special fractures of the hand (the **three B's—Bennett's, Boxer's,** and the **Baseball** fracture). **Bennett's fracture** is an intraarticular fracture of the base of the thumb metacarpal. A portion of the joint remains attached to the index metacarpal, and the remainder is dislocated. This injury will need surgical treatment but not urgently. Put the hand in a generous bulky dressing and send the patient to a hand specialist. **Boxer's fracture** is any impacted fracture of the head of the little-finger metacarpal (Figure 19-1A) secondary to a direct blow with a closed fist. Considerable angular deformity does not interfere with hand function (Figure 19-1B). Here, too, a bulky dressing and referral are appropriate. Up to 40° of angulation is acceptable. It is important to check for rotational deformities. A **baseball fracture** is an avulsion of the extensor tendon insertion from the base of the distal phalanx of a finger. Since the distal phalanx cannot extend (**mallet finger**), there is a reciprocal hyperextension of the proximal interphalangeal joint—the deformity of the whole finger is called **swan-neck deformity.** Splint the finger in extension. Depending on the size of the avulsed bone fragment (there may be none), surgical pinning may be indicated.

The universal bulky hand dressing consists of unfolded sponges that are placed loosely between the fingers so as not to occlude circulation and held on with a bandage. Try to hold the metacarpal-phalangeal joints in flexion and the interphalangeal joints in extension with the web space of the thumb open (the bye-bye baby position). A triangular bandage that positions the hand above the heart controls swelling.

Outpatient surgery to pin, plate, or externally fix a fracture can be done just as well three to five days after injury as immediately. However, compound fractures and joint wounds, as well as irreducible dislocations, need immediate attention.

SOFT TISSUE INJURIES OF THE HAND

Soft tissue injuries include damage to the ligaments and special structures around joints (sprains) and tendon lacerations

FIGURE 19-1 *A.* Angulated and slightly impacted fracture of the little-finger metacarpal head in a 20-year-old college student who hit a wall with his hand.

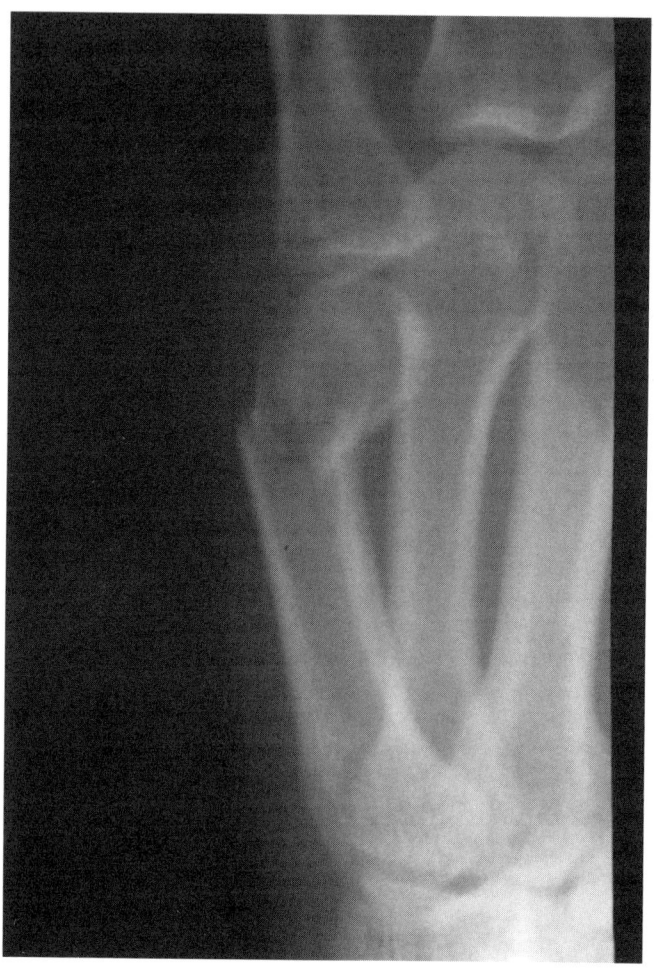

Hand Fractures and Soft Tissue Injuries 99

FIGURE 19-1 *(Continued) B.* After six weeks of treatment (a soft dressing for two weeks) he had full function. The metacarpal head is less prominent.

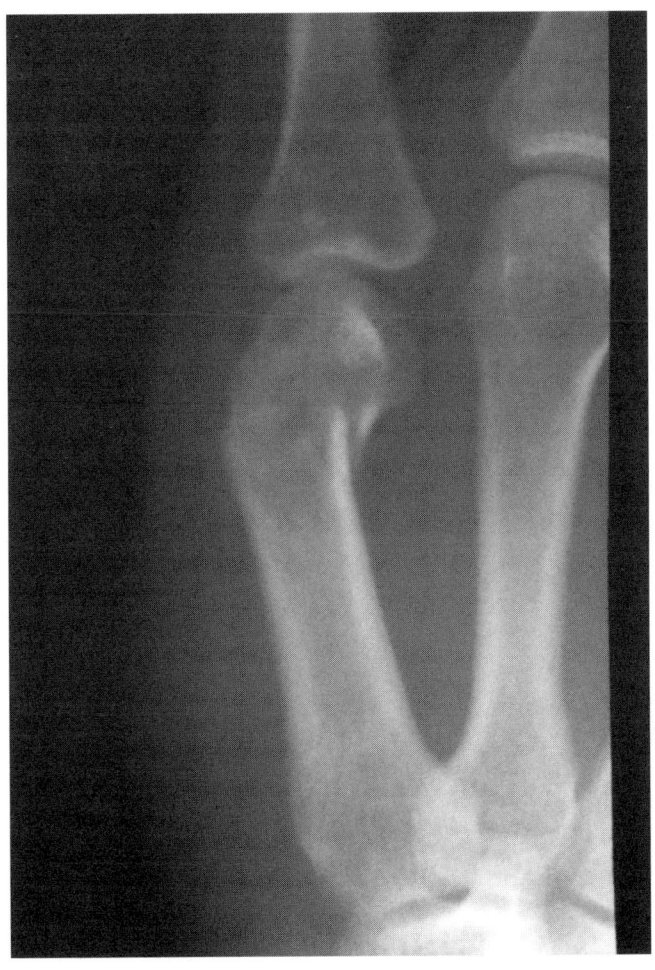

(strains). When a finger gets caught and is bent or twisted, often a swollen proximal interphalangeal joint results. This is a sprain of either the collateral ligaments that provide medial-lateral stability or of the volar plate. The plate keeps the middle phalanx from translating dorsally yet allows the fingers to bend. A radiograph may show that a sliver of bone has pulled off with the ligament (often called an avulsion fracture). A common fracture occurs at the metacarpal phalangeal joint of the thumb when it is wrenched by a ski-pole strap—skier's thumb. With the thumb straight, pull the thumb away from the hand—the ulnar collateral ligament should be taut. If it is lax, the thumb needs to be splinted, and repair may be required.

Tendon injuries can be divided into flexor and extensor types. The extensor lacerations on the dorsum of the hand are common and often uncomplicated. The easy ones can be blocked with local infiltration anesthesia and repaired with a few simple sutures in the ER. Close the skin loosely and apply a pressure dressing. The skin on the back of the hand is loose, and therefore a hematoma can accumulate easily. Splint the wrist and finger in extension

How do you know which ones are "easy"? Fair enough! Does the laceration go into the joint?—not so easy. Is there an associated compound fracture?—not easy. Extensive soft tissue wound?—and so on. If there is a large volume of cases and good organization, it is always better to work in an OR, where you will have good light, good instruments, and good help.

The **mallet finger** is really an extensor tendon strain and can have a large fracture from the base of the distal phalanx. Another extensor tendon injury is loss of the central portion of the extensor tendon as it passess over the PIP joint. Then the joint buttonholes the extensor mechanism, and a **boutonniere deformity** (flexion of the PIP joint) results. This is just the reciprocal of the swan-neck deformity, for now the distal phalanx extends.

Flexion tendon injuries are more exacting. They can be identified clinically because the position of the injured finger differs from the others; i.e., it sticks out when the other fingers are flexed. Support the PIP joint in extension and ask the patient to bend the fingertip—this checks the function of the long flexor. Hold the adjacent finger extended and ask the patient to flex the injured finger. If the PIP joint does not bend, than the sublimis tendon is torn. The profundus tendon to each finger runs through the sublimis tendon in a complex sheath, which begins at the metacarpal head and ends at the sublimis insertion in the middle phalanx. This used to be called "no man's land" because of the difficulty in repairing a tendon in this zone. Since the end of the finger is Zone I, this is now Zone II. Zone III is the palm. Zone IV is the area over the transverse carpal ligament. Zone V extends from transverse carpal ligament proximally. All flexor tendon injuries need surgical treatment in an operating room under magnification. A hand-surgery consult is necessary.

Chapter 20
Pelvic and Acetabular Fractures

In young patients, pelvic fracture occurs with severe high-speed traffic accidents. Old patients with diminished bone quality (osteoporosis) can trip on a rug at home, land on the buttocks, and sustain a pelvic fracture. All pelvic fractures are important. These fractures should be identified in the emergency room. The patient requires hospitalization to observe for internal injury—particularly *hemorrhage*.

Fractures of the *pelvic ring* differ from fractures of the acetabulum. Pelvic ring fractures can cause life-threatening hemorrhage, whereas acetabular fractures do not. Clinical signs of pelvic and acetabular fractures include asymmetry of the legs, pain in the pelvis, pain on hip motion, and—with anterior pelvic fractures—swelling and local tenderness at the symphysis. The diagnosis of pelvic fracture can almost always be made on plain x-ray of the pelvis if you know what to look for! Compare the pelvic inlet on both sides and look for fractures. Check the sacroiliac joints to see if one is wider. The sacral foraminae look like cat's eyes—the brows should be the same on both sides. The acetabular roof must be intact. (See Figure 20-1.) CT scan confirms the diagnosis and reveals and defines the fracture pattern. If a polytrauma patient must have a CT of the head, it is usually possible to get a pelvic CT at the same time. The CT is helpful in planning treatment.

FIGURE 20-1   The pelvic x-ray. A patient with a suspected pelvic fracture needs to have AP, inlet, and outlet view of the pelvis taken. The AP x-ray is depicted here. Check the symphysis pubis for widening or displacement. Also evaluate it for pubic rami fractures. As the pelvis is a complete circle, a fracture at one site must be accompanied by a second fracture site or area of disruption. Check the sacroiliac joints for widening and compare the sacral foramina. The foramina should be round. If an acetabular fracture is suspected, obtain Judet views. The iliac view is useful for visualizing the anterior rim of the acetabulum. Two useful lines that can be drawn on the AP x-ray are (1) iliopectineal line and (2) ilioischial line. If either of these lines does not have a smooth contour, this indicates a fracture.

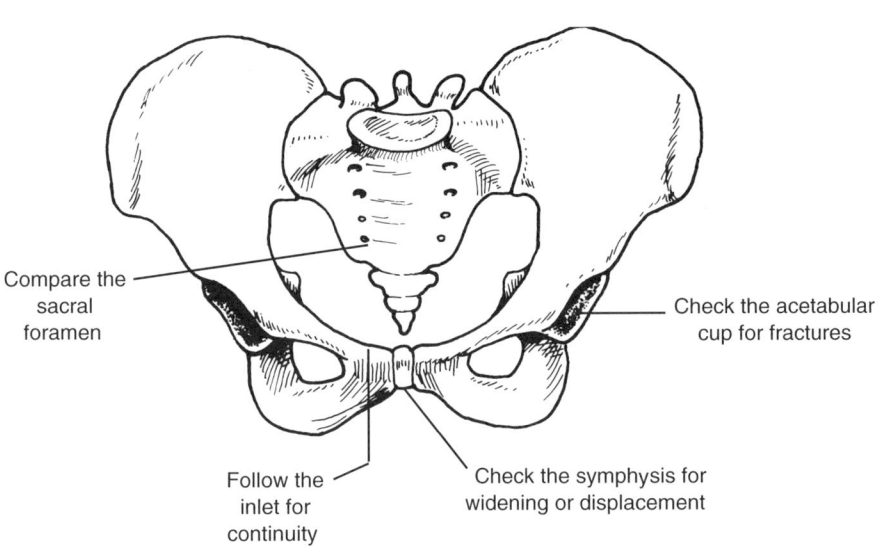

Initial emergency room care consists of splinting with a traction splint to control painful motion and reduce bleeding. A few sandbags or IV bags around the limb also help. Acetabular fractures are seldom operated on immediately: the procedure is planned for a few days after injury. Pelvic ring fractures with separation can be life threatening and need immediate attention if the patient is hemorrhaging.

The pelvis is a closed ring joined at the symphysis and sacroiliac joints. The ring must always break in two places. It is axiomatic, then, that a fracture of the pelvis is accompanied by either a sacral fracture or by a sacroiliac sprain. When the pelvis is fractured "front and back" on the same side, the combination is called Malgaigne's fracture. The name honors J. F. Malgaigne, the great Parisian surgeon who began the systematic study of fractured bones in the nineteenth century. When the ring opens, it can fill with blood. Therefore, all patients require intravenous access, a hematocrit, and or hemoglobin, prothrombin time and type and screen early in their emergency assessment. The further workup for displaced fractures includes an IVP, cystogram, and voiding cystourethrogram.

Measures that control bleeding include surgery to close the ring, angiography to embolize bleeding vessels, and compression garments (**MAST** trousers) to tamponade the bleeding. It may be possible to place pins and a clamp (external fixation) on the pelvis in the emergency room to control bleeding in a pelvis with associated hemorrhage (Figure 20-2A and B).

FIGURE 20-2 *A.* Initial pelvic film after accident shows separation of the symphysis anteriorly and disruption of the right sacroiliac joint with vertical translation of the whole right hemipelvis.

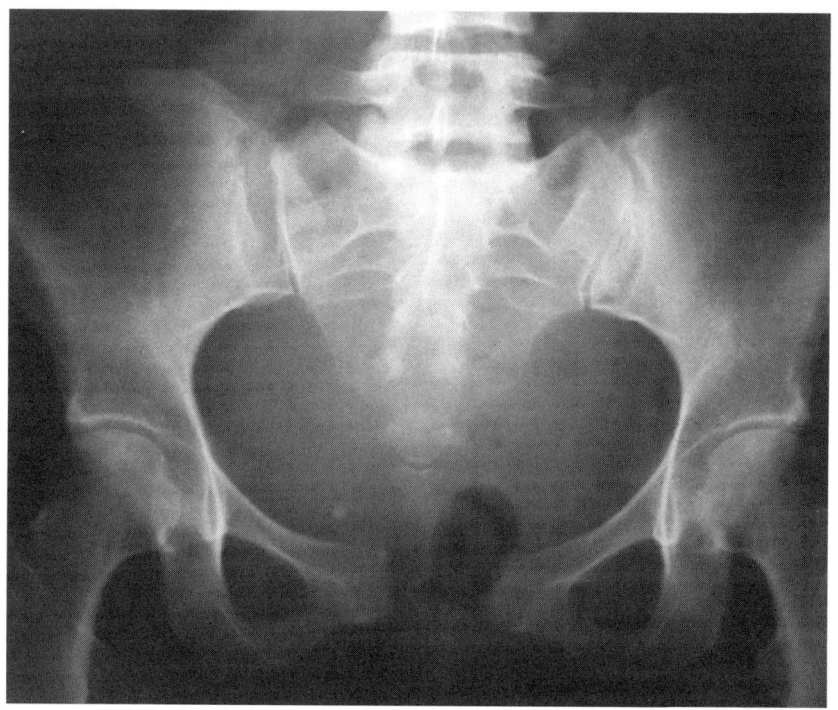

FIGURE 20-2 *(Continued)* **B.** Both components were stabilized to close the pelvic ring, control bleeding, and restore anatomy.

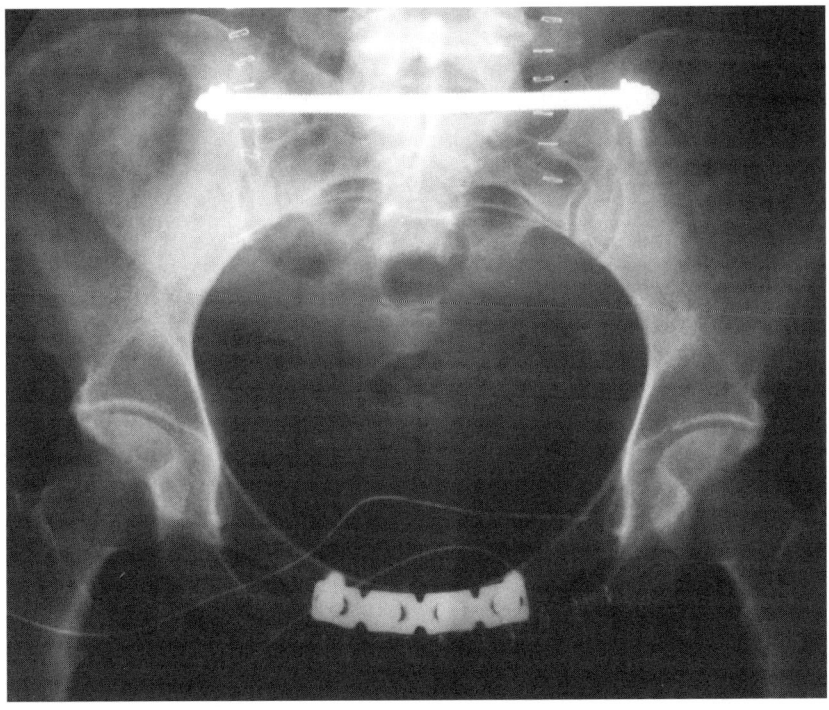

Chapter 21

Hip Fractures and Dislocations

The spectrum of emergent hip problems changes with age. Infants and children are subject to infections, dysplasia, and congenital dislocation; school children have osteonecrosis (Perthes' disease); adolescents have slipped capital femoral epiphysis; young adults suffer dislocations and complex high-energy fractures, and the elderly fall and have hip fractures.

There are common features to the clinical presentation. There is pain in the groin and inability to walk. The knee may hurt because the femoral nerve runs in proximity to the hip joint. The hip may be held in flexion to relax the femoral capsule. With fractures there is deformity, often with shortening and external rotation of the leg.

Place your hand on the knee and try to roll the hip internally and externally (like rolling dough for making bread). The affected hip will not roll smoothly—there will be "hip grab" on "log rolling." The evaluation will require at least a hematocrit & hemoglobin, WBC, and a plain x-ray that shows both hips. The "AP hips and pelvis" is a useful view that allows comparison of both hip joints. Sometimes the only finding will be an increase in the cartilage space when both hip joints are compared.

Hip pain always has an explanation. After an accident, pain in the hip is a fracture until proven otherwise. Observation in the hospital for more intensive investigation, such as a bone scan or tomography, is appropriate when the diagnosis cannot be excluded. Atraumatic hip pain in a child is an infection until proven otherwise. These diagnoses are too important to miss. See Figure 21-1 for an algorithm outlining basic diagnoses and treatment for hip pain.

A. HIP FRACTURES

Hip fractures occur in two different situations—falls in the elderly and as part of violent polytrauma of the young. In older patients, hip fractures are a common sign of frailty and decline and are a major cause of hospitalization (Figure 21-2A, B). Outcome depends a great deal on the preinjury level of function of the patient. In general, community ambulators return home, perhaps now using a cane or walker. Patients who arrive in the ER wearing slippers do not fare as well as a rule.

The x-ray identifies two basic fracture patterns—extracapsular and intracapsular fractures. Early recognition of the fracture type helps the orthopedist plan treatment, which is almost always operative. The intracapsular fracture is described as subcapital if the femoral head is broken off, like the cap of a mushroom off its stem, or transcervical if the fracture line is across the neck of the femur. The fracture at the base of the neck, which is like picking a mushroom with its stem, is a basicervical fracture. All these fractures are either displaced, nondisplaced, or impacted (driven together). To make this distiction a real true lateral x-ray must be taken. This can be done by flexing the uninjured leg over the x-ray tube and shooting across the table. A nondisplaced or impacted fracture can be treated with two or three percutaneously placed bone screws. A displaced fracture usually requires a femoral head replacement (Figure 21-2C). This operation is a greater one with considerable risk. It is important in the management of an elderly patient in the emergency department to avoid converting a nondisplaced fracture into a displaced one. This is best accomplished by minimizing manipulation of the leg. Placement of a skin traction boot with 2 kg (5 lb.) of traction

FIGURE 21-1 When a patient presents with a painful hip following an accident, x-rays (AP and lateral) of the hip should be obtained. If no fractures are evident, send the patient home on crutches and have them follow up in a couple of days. If a fracture is present, place the patient in traction, as the patient will require operative treatment. The type of fixation, however, is dependent on whether the fracture is intra- or extracapsular.

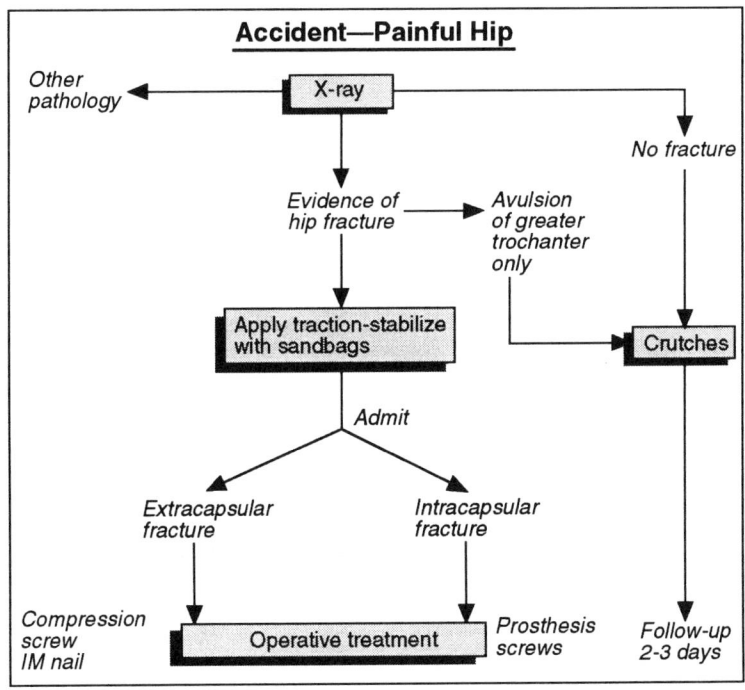

FIGURE 21-2 *A.* In this intracapsular fracture of the hip in a 68-year-old woman, note the intertrochanteric line is intact. There is shortening and displacement. In no view does the femoral head and neck appear as a gentle "S" curve.

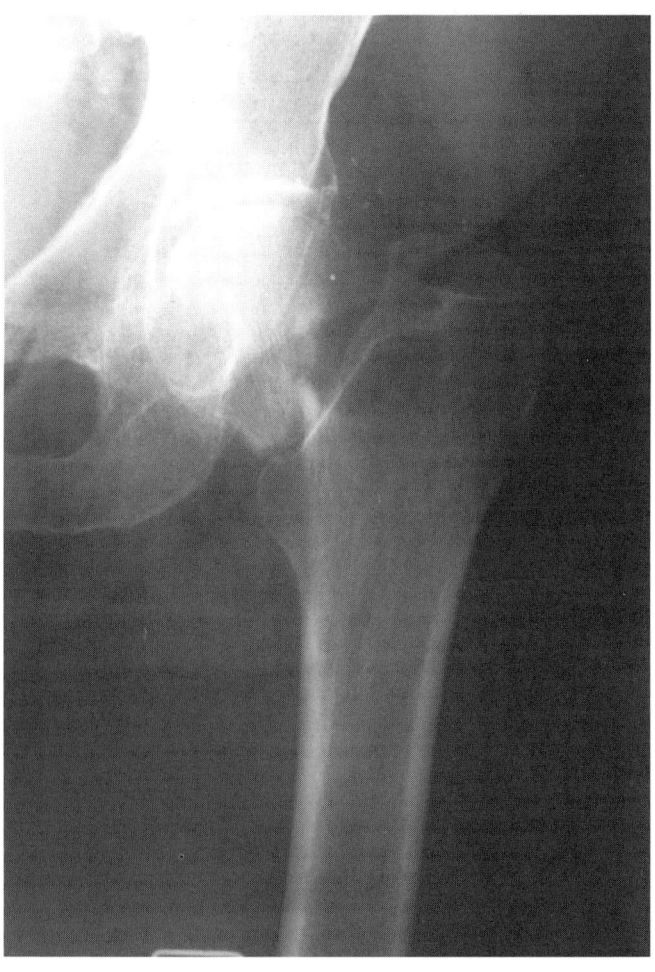

FIGURE 21-2 *(Continued) B.* **The lateral x-ray.**

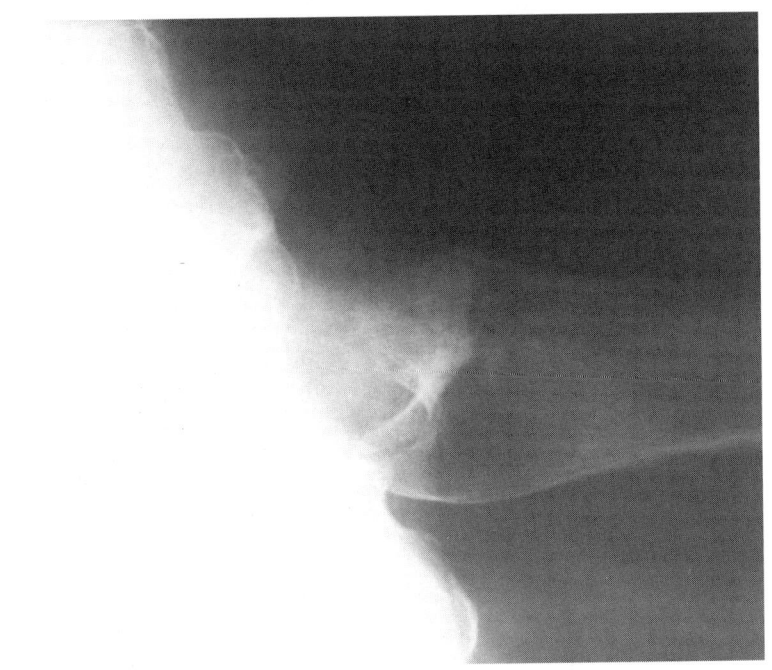

FIGURE 21-2 *(Continued)* C. The treatment was a multiple-part (bipolar) prosthesis.

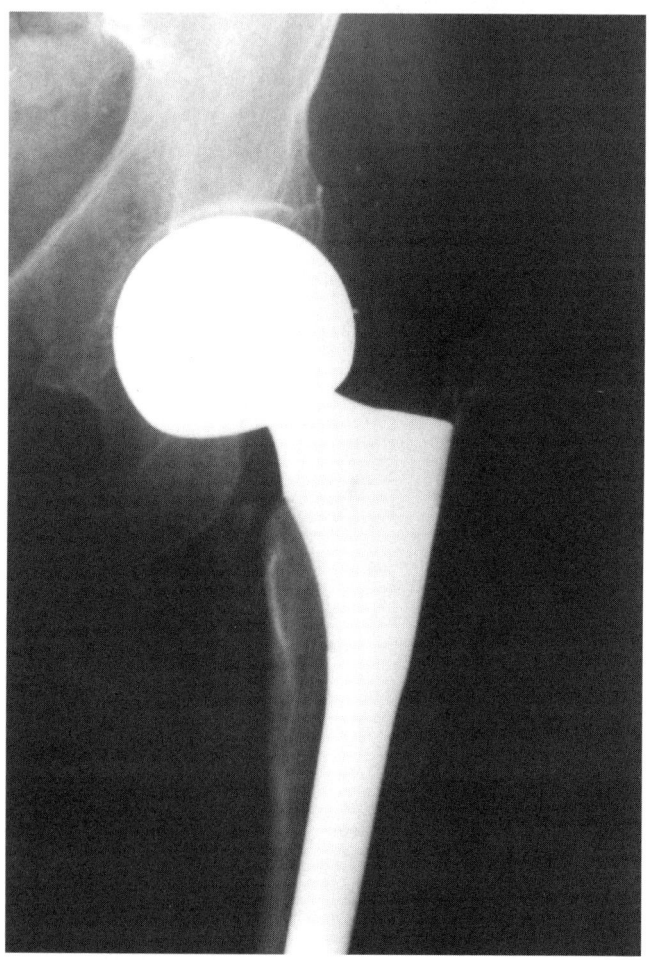

and placement of sandbags or plastic IV bottles around the thigh will control rotation.

The second major group of hip fractures in elderly patients are intertrochanteric fractures. These involve a fracture between the base of the neck and the lesser trochanter. The simplest fracture is one parallel to the intertrochanteric line. This is seen as a dense condensation of bone on the dorsal surface of the proximal femur, which on x-ray runs from the tip of the greater trochanter laterally and obliquely toward the lesser trochanter. The fracture line is seen as a sharp jagged line paralleling the intertrochanteric line that divides the proximal femur into two pieces—a "two-part intertrochanteric fracture." With more comminution there are more pieces. Do not confuse the head-neck fragment of a "four-part intertroch" with a basicervical fracture. Look along the intertrochanteric line and at the trochanters and find the rest of the fracture that makes this a true intertrochanteric fracture. (See Figure 21-3.)

Extracapsular fractures are generally treated with either sliding screw plate devices or intramedullary nails. Hip fractures and dislocations in patients under 60 are often atypical and challenging to repair and may be the source of long-term disability. The patterns are not comparable to the ones observed in the elderly. Fractures distal to the lesser trochanter are more frequent. These are called "subtrochanteric fractures." Since the stress in the femur is highest in this area, fixation that does not fail prior to fracture healing is more difficult to achieve. Late implant breakage is not uncommon. It is helpful when talking to families to be able to distinguish the types of hip fracture and indicate the difficulties of their probable treatment. Elderly patients are at risk because of their diminished physiological reserve for major surgery. Young patients have high mechanical demands and complex fractures.

Some common problems that present back to the ER in elderly patients after hip-fracture fixation are given in Table 21-1.

FIGURE 21-3 The signs of hip fracture.

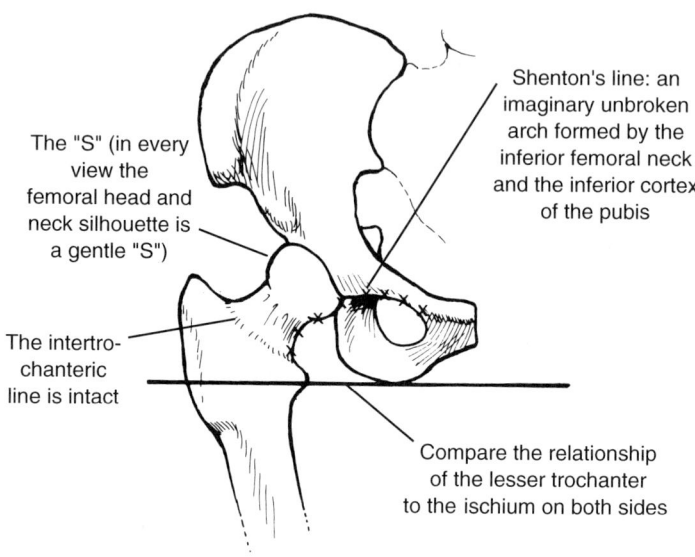

TABLE 21-1 Common Problems Following Hip-Fracture Fixation in the Elderly

PROBLEM	CAUSE	CONFIRMED BY
Swollen leg	Thrombophlebitis	Venous Doppler
Painful trochanter	Prominent screws	Plain x-rays
Short leg	Dislocated prosthesis	Plain x-rays
Groin pain	Osteonecrosis	Bone scan

B. HIP DISLOCATIONS

In adults, hip dislocations occur in major motor vehicle accidents. Most commonly the knee strikes the dashboard and forces the femoral head out the back of the hip socket. Most hip dislocations are posterior, because the hip socket faces somewhat anteriorly, allowing the femoral head to strike the posterior lip of the acetabulum and dislocate. If you understand this mechanism, you will understand how fractures of the posterior acetabular wall or femoral head occur with dislocations and how fragments come to lie in the hip joint after it is reduced.

Clinically the leg is shortened, internally rotated, and painful. Minutes after dislocation, reduction is often possible by simply pulling on the leg. As minutes become hours, muscle tension increases and maintains the dislocation, and reduction is progressively more difficult. There are several classic methods for replacing a hip dislocation. For example, with the patient on the floor, traction and flexion of the hip toward the opposite shoulder sometimes works. Unless you are stuck on an expedition in a medically impoverished country, it is sensible to try to reduce the hip with traction and some sedation in the ER, and, if a reduction cannot be achieved, to try under general anesthesia with paralysis or with a spinal anesthetic.

Open reduction will be necessary if a large fragment prevents the femoral head from seating in the acetabulum, if the femoral head is impacted on the acetabulum lip, or in atypical dislocations where closed reduction is not successful.

The sequence for managing a hip dislocation has to be individualized. Several points are worth remembering:

1. Hip dislocations are painful.
2. The longer the hip is dislocated, the greater the risk of death of the femoral head (osteonecrosis).
3. Most patients need a CT scan to evaluate the joint for fragments.
4. Unstable hips (i.e., ones that dislocate after reduction) are associated with large posterior lip fragments.

However, a dislocated hip is not in as desperate straits as a fish out of water. The incidence of osteonecrosis is not great in the first twelve hours, so there is time for workup. Individualize care! If the patient is given succinyl choline for intubation, that is a good moment to reduce the hip with in-line traction. If a patient must go to CT for a head injury, get a few cuts through the hip joint.

Adults with hip dislocations are generally placed in skeletal traction after reduction. The pin is usually inserted in the distal femur. Traction controls the rotation of the thigh and distracts the joint. It overcomes painful muscle spasm. Traction prevents redislocation of the hip.

In children, a painful hip always requires an explanation. The child presents with limping or outright refusal to walk. This is never a psychological problem. Review a good AP x-ray of the hips and pelvis with a radiologist and remember to look for the common conditions. In a child, a hip with fluid should be aspirated if sepsis cannot be ruled out. Toxic synovitis is a benign postviral effusion in the hip. The child is not febrile. The systemic white count is not elevated. The child is placed in skin traction under observation. Symptoms resolve slowly; with sepsis they worsen.

In adolescent boys, limping after a minor fall may represent slipped capital femoral epiphysis. This diagnosis is made clinically by loss of external rotation in the affected hip and on x-ray by the seating of the femoral head on the femoral neck. Review the findings with a radiologist and compare with illustrations in an atlas. A slipped epiphysis need to be pinned.

Chapter 22
Femoral Shaft Fractures

Femur fractures occur most frequently in young adults involved in motor vehicle accidents or other high-energy trauma. The fractures are commonly displaced because of the action of large muscle groups on the fragments. The usual presentation is a patient with an obviously deformed thigh, pain, and inability to walk. These patients are placed in traction splints (e.g., a Thomas splint) to avoid muscle damage from jagged bone ends and to make the patient more comfortable. The splint should be left in place until the patient is placed in skeletal traction or operatively stabilized. In adults, these injuries are mostly treated with intramedullary nailing.

Because femur fractures are associated with high-energy acccidents, a thorough evaluation must be performed. Vital signs are important, as femur fractures are frequently associated with shock and fat embolism, as well as neurovascular compromise. Examine the thigh for open wounds. Assess dorsalis pedis and posterior tibial pulses, capillary refill, and the patient's ability to dorsiflex and plantarflex the foot. Nerve injuries are uncommon because of the protection afforded to the nerve by the surrounding soft tissue. Patients with neurovascular compromise need immediate attention. Be aware of a hematoma that is expanding or a diminishing pulse, as these may be signs of an arterial injury. Arteriography is indicated if arterial injury is suspected. Ligamentous injuries at the knee and patella fractures are not uncommon in femoral shaft fractures; a hemarthrosis is one clue.

In the emergency room obtain at least a hemoglobin, hematocrit, prothrombin time, and blood type and screen. A femur fracture can be a cause of hemorrhagic shock. A femur fracture may result in at least a two-unit blood loss into the thigh. Obtain an arterial oxygen on room air and then place the patient on supplemental oxygen therapy. The baseline arterial oxygen is important for planning treatment of the fracture as well as for determining the patient's immediate needs. Always secure an adequate intravenous line. Polytrauma patients require a Foley catheter to measure output. Finally, check the splinting to be sure that there is not excess pressure in the groin, on the sciatic nerve in the gluteal crease, on the popliteal vessels behind the knee, on the peroneal nerve as it winds around the proximal fibula, or on the dorsum of the foot or on the heel.

Anterposterior and lateral x-rays of the femur, hip, knee, and tibia should be obtained. The x-ray workup must show not only the fracture but also two good views of the hip and knee, since there is an association between femur shaft fractures and fractures of the hip and the knee. A nondisplaced hip fracture can become displaced during intramedullary nailing of a femur shaft if it is not detected and properly repaired. Another association is the presence of an ipsilateral tibia fracture resulting in a condition known as a **floating knee**—so named because both a femur fracture and a tibia fracture exist in the same extremity, making the knee a free-floating entity. The fracture pattern (spiral, oblique, transverse), complexity (simple, comminuted, complex comminuted), and location (proximal, middle, distal third) are described from the x-ray (Figure 22-1). Long spiral fractures are occasionally seen after seemingly minor twisting falls. Transverse fractures are the result of impact and bending.

The emergent treatment of femoral shaft fractures is important in that it stabilizes the fracture and allows for early mobilization, both of which aid in decreasing the mortality and morbidity (by decreasing blood loss and the incidence of fat embolism and pneumonia) associated with femoral shaft fractures. The usual treatment choice is closed intramedullary nailing. The presence of an open wound, se-

FIGURE 22-1 This fracture is the subtrochanteric region, because it involves the femur distal to the lesser trochanter. The basic type is spiral, because the fracture line twists around the femur. This is a comminuted fracture with a large butterfly fragment containing the lesser trochanter.

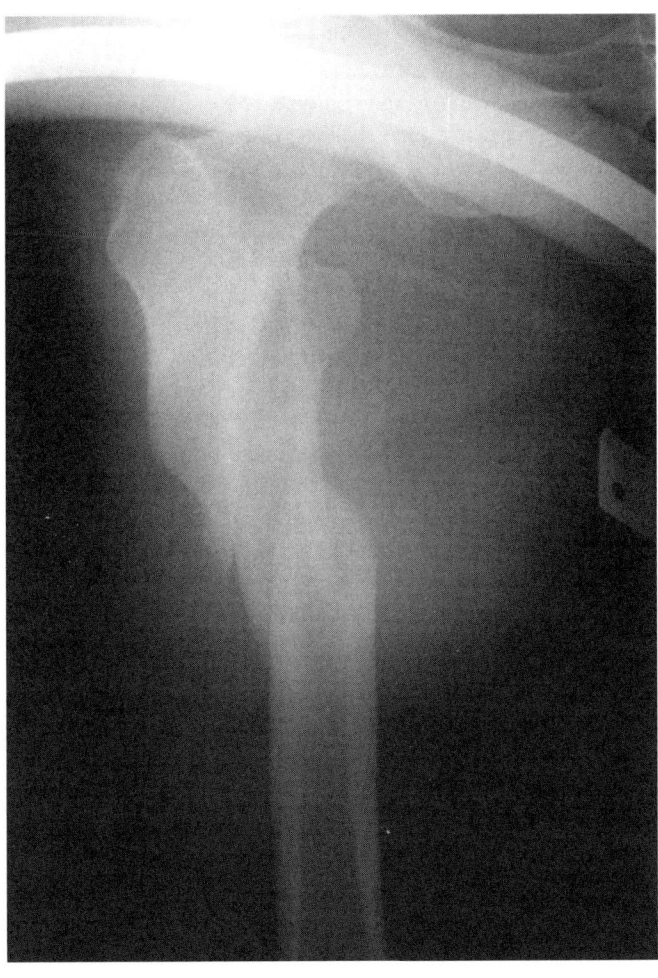

vere comminution, or other complicating factors may require an alternative method of fixation.

Timing is important. A femur shaft fracture invariably reduces oxygenation in the days following injury. When the reduction is profound, the condition is called fat embolism syndrome. Placement of a nail lengthwise in the marrow cavity (intramedullary nailing) also reduces oxygenation. These two effects can be additive. Therefore, the baseline room-air arterial gas should be monitored to determine when it is safe to nail the bone. Nailing can be safely performed on the day of injury if the room-air arterial oxygen is over 80 mm Hg. Following that, it is advisable to wait until the postfracture depression in oxygenation has bottomed out and begins to return toward normal.

Common problems in patients discharged from the hospital after a femur fracture are swollen leg from thrombophlebitis and chest pain and/or tachypnea from pulmonary embolism. There may be swelling over the trochanter from a postoperative hematoma and pain over the sites of screws that are placed through the nail to maintain length and rotation. A change in the shape of the thigh indicates implant failure—take an x-ray.

Fat embolism syndrome is a full-blown complication of femur fractures. Transportation over long distances without splinting increases its incidence. The hallmarks are hypoxia, petechiae, tachypnea, and neurological dysfunction. The diagnosis of fat embolism is made by the above findings in addition to a low PO_2 (usually less than 60 mm Hg). Fat globules can be found in the urine. Look for the presence of radiographic changes on chest x-ray (usually after first 24 hours). Oxygen by nasal prongs or mask is helpful in protecting the lungs from fat embolism. Treatment of fat embolism consists of ventilatory support with the use of PEEP (positive end expiratory pressure).

Chapter 23
Injuries about the Knee

A. KNEE INJURIES

The knee is vulnerable. Whether checked or blocked on the playing field at sports, driven into the dashboard in an accident, or struck on the road during a motorcycle accident, knees are subject to fracture and complex injury.

Mechanically, the knee joint is a rolling cam. It does not just bend like a simple hinge, but rather the tibia translates posteriorly as the knee flexes. Anterior-posterior stability through the arc of motion is maintained by the anterior and posterior cruciate ligaments. Remember that the **anterior cruciate ligament** keeps the tibia from translating anteriorly in relation to the distal femur and the **posterior cruciate ligament** keeps the tibia from falling posterior.

The position the knee was injured in may be different from the one in which it is examined. An ATV driver who injures the knee in the seated position with the knee flexed may be evaluated on a stretcher with the knee in the straight-neutral position. To do a good job, always have the patient undressed from thigh to toes on both sides. The uninjured knee serves as the control. Tight shorts need to come off, because they will restrict the quadriceps. The examination depends on following a specific routine to evaluate the soft tissue structures in turn. It is better to find a displaced fracture of the medial femoral condyle on the x-ray before you manipulate the knee.

Learn a little bit more each time you examine a patient with a knee injury. This is a complex joint essential for comfortable bipedal function, and it will take a while to develop the skills you need to evaluate the knee properly.

B. FRACTURES OF THE DISTAL FEMUR AND PROXIMAL TIBIA

After a motor vehicle accident, patients with significant fractures about the knee usually have evident clinical deformity. In the distal femur these often high-energy fractures are called **supracondylar fractures,** and in the proximal tibia they are metaphyseal fractures of the proximal tibia.

Since the neurovascular structures are bound by fascia to the posterior surface of the joint, these patients are at high risk for vascular or neurologic injury. Begin by splinting the limb, and assess capillary flow and pulsatile circulation of the foot. Verify that the major divisions of the sciatic nerve are intact by having the patient dorsiflex the toes (peroneal nerve) and plantarflex the toes (posterior tibial nerve).

These injuries are generally easy to diagnose on x-ray. However, look carefully at the lateral x-ray of the distal femur to find fractures in the coronal plane. These, Hoffa fractures, are spotted by following the outline of the larger medial and smaller lateral distal femoral condyle. Check the intercondylar eminence. It keeps the condyles lined up on the tibial plateaus and can be fractured. Look at the clear space of the knee. If there are fragments, these should be triangulated in the other projection to determine their location. Loose pieces can come from either the femur or tibia with torn ligaments or detached menisci (**Segond fractures**).

Since patients with major fractures about the knee cannot ambulate and are at risk for compartment syndrome, they are admitted to the hospital for several days. When the joint surface is significantly displaced, internal fixation is indicated. Initially, traction will usually restore basic relationships, and then surgical reconstruction can be performed on a semielective basis.

Always think about the potential that fractures of the distal femur and proximal tibia have for vascular injury. The extent of displacement at the moment of injury may be great and does not necessarily correspond to the position at the time x-rays are taken. A steady pulse or good Doppler exam does not rule out occult intimal damage, which will become clinically manifest hours or days later. If in doubt, obtain an arteriogram.

Supracondylar and major proximal tibia fractures differ in their severity from **tibial plateau fractures**. Plateau fractures are common after falls in older patients who have osteoporotic bone (Figure 23-1A, B). In these cases deformity may be minimal and neurovascular injury is unlikely. Patients with plateau fractures are initially immobilized in a well-padded knee immobilizer. Tomography may help to demonstrate the depressed articular fracture or split, which is commonly in the lateral tibial plateau. Often the plateau is widened (split) and a joint fragment is driven into the proximal tibia (depressed).

Children sustain different patterns of injury. Fractures of the distal femur involve the growth plate. The more complex the injury, the greater the chance for growth disturbance. In the proximal femur and distal tibia are the most rapidly growing epiphyses of the lower limb (Figure 23-2). Unusual skeletal conditions therefore tend to localize about the knee. Two common findings should not be confused with significant skeletal pathology or fractures. These are painful apophysitis of the tibial tubercle in growing boys (**Osgood-Schlatter's disease**) and posttraumatic calcification of the medial collateral ligament (**Pelligrini-Steada disease**). These findings have been inappropriately named "diseases" to the increased concern of parents everywhere.

FIGURE 23-1 *A.* This 51-year old nurse anesthetist with rheumatoid arthritis fell and fractured her distal femur. The bone is markedly osteoporotic.

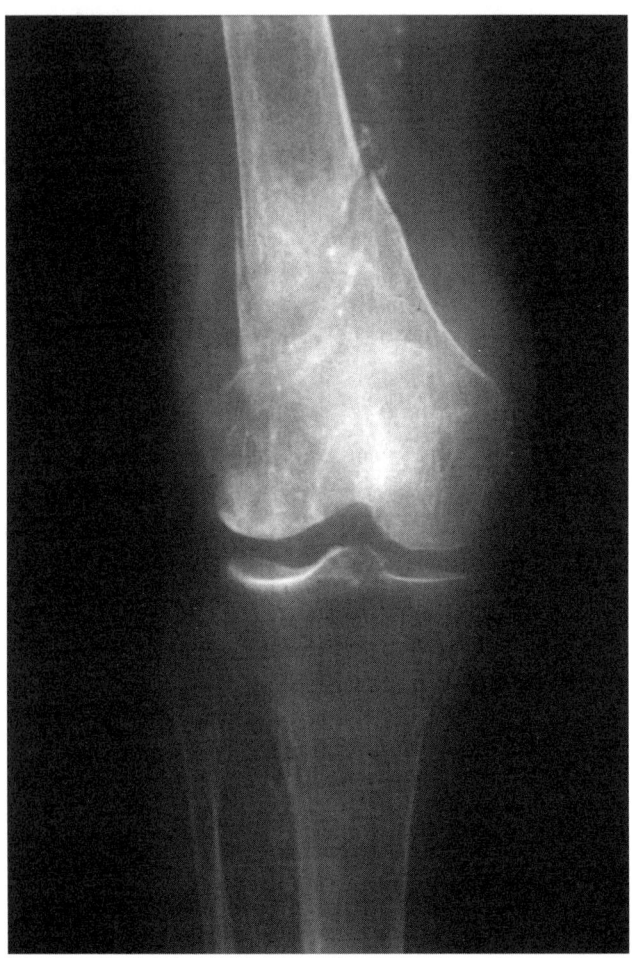

FIGURE 23-1 *(Continued)* **B. Internal fixation was required. All supracondylar fractures will need initially to be hospitalized.**

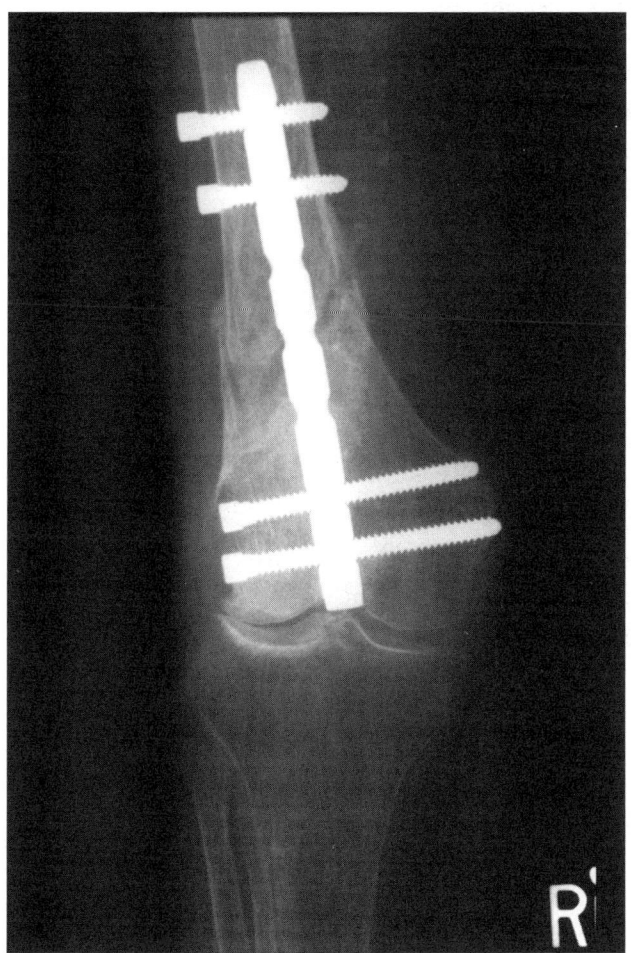

FIGURE 23-2 Pediatric epiphyseal injuries. Epiphyseal slips as studied by Pollard of Boston carry a small triangle of metaphyseal bone. An easy mnemonic for remembering the classification of these, SALTeR (as modified by Salter of Toronto), is as follows:

S—Same level as epiphyseal plate
A—Above the level of the epiphyseal plate
L—Lower than the level of the epiphyseal plate
T—Through the epiphyseal plate
e
R—cRush

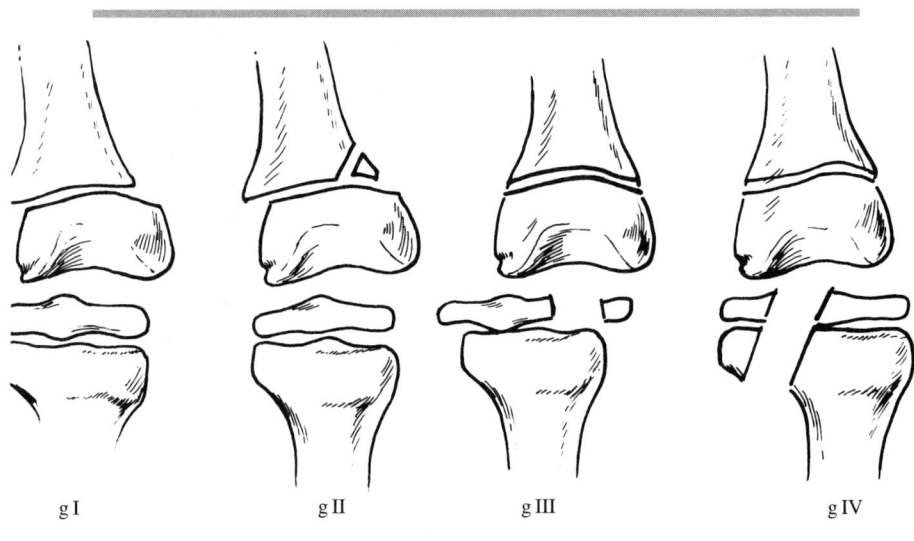

g I
Epiphyseal slip

g II
Epiphyseal slip with metaphyseal fragment

g III
Trans-epiphyseal fracture

g IV
Epiphyseal-diaphyseal fracture

C. PATELLA FRACTURES

The knee cap, or patella, increases the efficiency of the quadriceps muscles by offsetting its pull from the axis of rotation of the knee. Unfortunately, the patella often strikes the dashboard or the pavement and is frequently fractured. On examination, note the position of the patella. Inspect the knee for swelling and ecchymosis. Determine if there is tenderness and crepitus by palpating the patella. Palpate the soft tissue for defects and put the knee through both passive and active range of motion. The diagnosis of patella fracture when there are several widely separated fragments is straightforward. However, a nondisplaced fracture can be confused with an incompletely formed patella, known as a bipartite patella (Figure 23-3.) Correlation of the clinical examination with the x-ray findings (acute fractures are sharp discontinuities without rounded, reactive margins) usually clarifies the diagnosis. In addition, a bipartite patella usually involves the superior and lateral quadrant of the patella. Nondisplaced fractures are splinted with the knee in extension, while displaced fractures greater than 4 mm are taken to the operating room for reduction and fixation. Extremely comminuted fractures of the patella can be excised. Note that if the retinaculum on both sides of the patella is intact, the patient will be able to set the knee and raise the leg, even if the patella is fractured.

Ruptures of the central slip of the quadriceps or of the patellar tendon are uncommon. They can be diagnosed by a gap in the soft tissues above or below the patella on examination and an unusually superior or inferior position of the patella on x-ray. On the lateral x-ray with the knee in some flexion the patella lies between the distal femoral epiphyseal scars. A high-riding patella is called **patella alta** and a low-riding patella **patella baja**. These are the **a**'s and **b**'s of patella position.

The tracking of the patella across the anterior face of the distal femur is a precise mechanism that is easily damaged. The patella can sublux or dislocate laterally. When the patella slips laterally, the medial structures must be torn. Therefore, when the patella is relocated, tenderness in the retinaculum is medial to the patella and apprehension when the patella is

FIGURE 23-3 Extensor mechanism of the knee. The patella plays a crucial role in the extensor mechanism, as it increases the lever arm of the quadriceps muscle, thereby decreasing the force necessary to extend the tibia. The patella tendon attaches the quadriceps to the tibial tubercle. The patella is encased in the tendon and is thus known as a sesmoid bone—the largest in the body. A bipartite patella is a common anomaly and is often misdiagnosed as a fracture. It is often located in the superior pole of the patella.

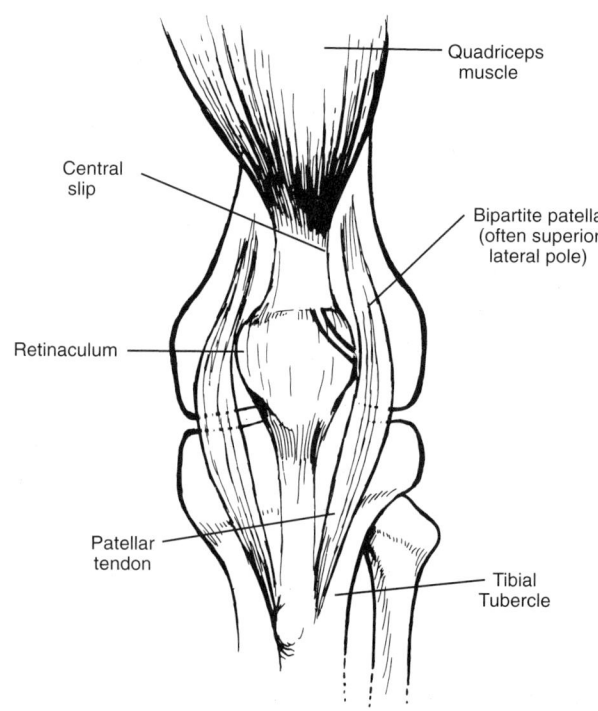

shifted laterally by the examiner are the signs of the injury. Many patients call a dislocated patella a "dislocated knee." Be sure to make the distinction. Contusions to the knee can produce distressing subpatellar symptoms or infrapatellar fat pad swelling. A small bursa overlying the patella can fill with fluid, particularly after repetitive trauma. Working people who must be down on their knees, e.g., carpenters or carpet layers, are susceptible to this condition. When marked inflammation is present, the bursa should be aspirated with a large-bore needle and a specimen sent for culture. The patient should then be started on antibiotics.

LIGAMENTOUS INJURIES OF THE KNEE AND KNEE DISLOCATIONS

Significant soft tissue injuries of the knee are an important diagnostic puzzle in young, active adults. Triage is directed toward detecting new injury, preventing damage, and setting the stage for recovery. There are three paired structures to consider, given in Table 23-1. In each pair, injury to the first structure is much more likely than to the second. Time after injury changes the examination. Shortly following an accident there is no effusion, little pain, and no muscle spasm. The evaluation for stability can be easily conducted. Experienced examiners can assess ligaments with great accuracy right on the football field. The evaluation becomes more difficult with the passage of time. Before examining the individual, it is important to determine the mechanism of injury.

TABLE 23-1 Soft Tissues of the Knee

STRUCTURE	FUNCTION
Medial/lateral meniscus	Load transfer
anterior/posterior cruciate ligaments	AP stability
Medial/lateral collateral ligaments	Varus-valgus stability

Knowing this, one can often determine what physical findings to expect. It is also important to know if the patient has had previous knee injuries.

Inspect the knee for atrophy, swelling, and deformity. Palpate the knee, feeling for deformity and crepitus. Determine areas of tenderness. Next put the knee through gentle passive range of motion (Figure 23-4).

FIGURE 23-4 Accident—painful knee. In the patient who suffers a knee injury, the initial evaluation should include a thorough examination and x-rays (AP and lateral). The exam, however, will dictate whether views of the patella are necessary. The most useful view of the patella is the Merchant view, obtained with the knees in 45° of flexion and the x-ray beam directed toward the feet. If, on exam, pulses are undetectable, or if vascular injury is suspected, an emergent arteriogram is necessary. If positive, obtain vascular consult and prepare the patient for surgery. Once vascular injury has been ruled out, x-rays should be examined for fracture or dislocation. If there is a fracture of the tibial metaphysis, an arteriogram should also be obtained to rule out vascular injury. If a fracture is present, place the patient in a long leg splint, evaluate the extremity and obtain orthopedic consult. The patient will probably need to be admitted. For patients who suffer nondisplaced fractures or grade I or II ligamentous sprains, the definitive treatment will be a closed cast. If the fracture is displaced or if there is a grade III ligamentous sprain, operative repair will be required. If the exam reveals instability, but the x-rays show no fracture or dislocation, suspect injury to one of the major stabilizing ligaments to the knee. Depending on the degree of instability, which ligament(s) is (are) affected, and the age and activity of the patient, operative repair may be necessary. The diagnosis of instability can be confirmed with arthroscopy of the knee joint. If the joint is stable, place the patient in a knee immobilizer and have the patient follow up in three to five days.

FIGURE 23-4 *(Continued)*

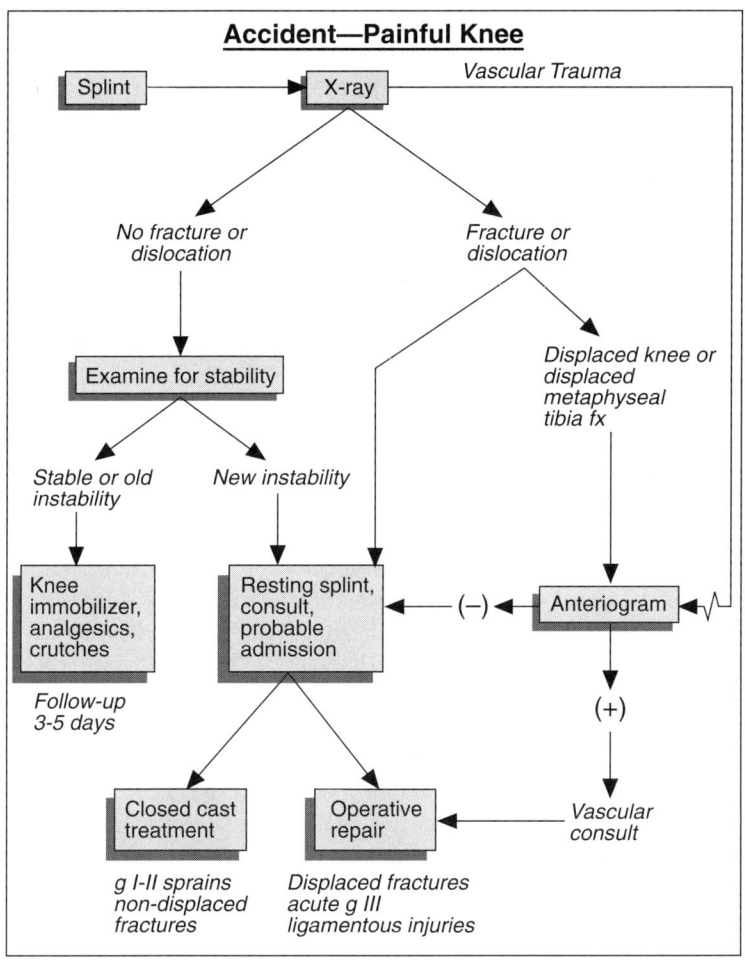

The anterior and posterior cruciate ligaments control AP stability of the knee. With the knee extended, the anterior cruciate prevents the tibia from translating anteriorly. The **Lachmann test** was designed to test the anterior cruciate ligament (ACL). The test is useful in patients with an acute injury. It is performed with the patient supine and the knee in 15–20° of flexion. One of the examiner's hands is placed on the distal femur, the other on the proximal tibia. Then an anteriorly directed force is applied to the proximal tibia by the examiner's hand. In a knee in which the ACL is disrupted, there will be no clear endpoint, and anterior translation is detected. This indicates a positive test.

The **anterior drawer test** is also useful to determine the integrity of the ACL. Once again, place the patient supine, flex the hip to approximately 45° and the knee to 90°. The foot should be flat on the examining table. Then, using both hands, apply an anteriorly directed force to the posterior aspect of the proximal tibia. A translation of 6–8 mm indicates a positive test.

Posterior cruciate ligament (PCL) injuries are uncommon. They occur mostly after high-speed motor vehicle When a PCL disruption is suspected, one should inspect the knee for a posterior sag indicating PCL laxity. The **posterior drawer test,** which is used to test the PCL, is performed with the patient in the same position as for the anterior drawer test. This time instead of applying an anterior force, a posteriorly directed force is applied to the anterior aspect of the proximal tibia. Lack of an endpoint indicates a positive test.

The collateral ligaments of the knee are its lateral and medial stabilizers. The more infrequent lateral collateral injuries are associated with fracture of the fibular head and peroneal nerve palsy. To test the medial collateral ligament have the patient sit at the end of the examining table with the affected leg in 20° of flexion. Then apply a laterally directed force to the ankle and a medially directed force to the proximal tibia. If the medial collateral ligament is disrupted, the knee joint will open on the medial side. The lateral collateral ligament is tested in much the same way, except that the direction of the forces is reversed, and the knee is extended.

Torn menisci cause symptoms of **internal derangement** of the knee. Internal derangement is a symptom complex that results from a loose component inside the joint; e.g., a bone or cartilage fragment, torn meniscus, etc. The three features of internal derangement are (1) **locking,** (2) "knee **giving** out," and (3) **recurrent effusion.** A locked knee is one that gets stuck in flexion and has to be twisted to "unlock" it. "Giving" means the patient experiences a sudden loss of support when using the leg. This is caused by reflex quadriceps inhibition: it is involuntary. Recurrent effusions usually occur after episodes of "locking" or "giving." When at least two of these three features are present along with tenderness over the meniscus at the joint line, the tender compartment most likely has a torn meniscus. **MacMurray's test** is used to test for meniscal tears. The test is performed by placing the patient supine, flexing the knee to be tested, and then externally rotating the tibia while simultaneously applying a valgus stress to the proximal tibia. The presence of clicking at the posterior joint line when rotating the flexed leg on the femur indicates a positive test and meniscal injury. The signs of chronic instability from torn collateral and cruciate ligaments are the same as those of the torn menisci. These symptoms develop in the weeks after acute untreated injury and are accompanied by quadriceps atrophy.

In most cases when isolated ligamentous tears are diagnosed, it is appropriate to wrap the knee in cast padding, apply a loose covering bandage (e.g., an ACE wrap) and a knee immobilizer, and arrange for follow-up with an orthopedist specializing in sports medicine within 48–72 hours. The patient will need crutches and analgesics. An ice pack applied to the outside of the dressing is probably not harmful and helps control pain.

Dislocation of the tibia is a severe injury that carries the risk of vascular injury (Figure 23-5). Reduction is an emergency and may require an anesthetic. The ligaments that must be torn depend on the direction of the dislocation. The importance of this injury should not be overlooked in a polytrauma patient where the initial reduction has been achieved during resuscitation. An arteriogram is often helpful in detecting occult arterial injury. The limb is at risk for compartment syndrome of the leg in the hours and days after reduc-

FIGURE 23-5 Dislocation of the knee. The tibia was driven posterior and laterally—the medial collateral and posterior cruciate ligaments were torn. Arteriogram shows occlusion of the superficial femoral artery with some reconstruction of the artery by collaterals.

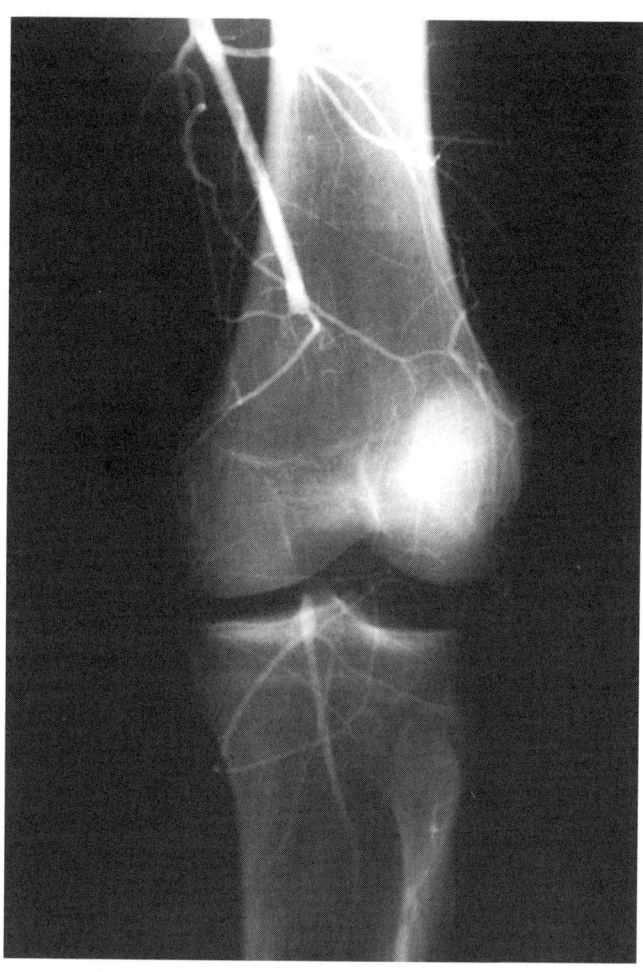

tion. A baseline measurement of compartment pressure is useful to obtain, particularly in unconscious patients. The pressure can be measured manometrically with a needle placed in the compartment. A hand-held device is also available. Compartment pressure should be followed in relation to mean arterial pressure. After reduction, the leg is placed in a bulky dressing from toes to thigh. Unlike the hip or shoulder, the reduction of the knee may not be concentric. This is because of the complex ligaments responsible for knee stability. Operative repair may be required in the days after injury. The results are usually far from perfect.

Chapter 24
Leg Fractures

A fractured tibia occurs most often in young adults as a consequence of motor vehicle accidents and sports injuries. If the fibula is also fractured, the combination is called a "tib-fib" fracture. The tibia, however, is the most important consideration, since it does most of the load-bearing work of the leg, and its length and alignment need to be restored as accurately as possible for full function. If the tibia is fractured, but the fracture is very nearly lined up, it can be successfully managed in a cast.

In the emergency department all care should be taken to assure that the leg with a fracture in an acceptable position can be treated nonoperatively. First the x-ray is taken in the splint. Then the cast is carefully applied. A fracture of the lower half of the tibial shaft can be treated in a cast that extends from the knee distal (**patellar tendon bearing cast (PTB)**), while a fracture of the upper tibial shaft is placed in a long leg cast. In general, the patient placed in a circular cast is admitted for 24- to 48-hour observation to be sure that the cast does not become too tight. In the hospital, the patient can be fitted with crutches and taught an appropriate gait. Patients usually require more than "overnight" observation, since swelling is maximal at 36 to 48 hours. (See Figure 24-1.)

Displaced fractures are a serious problem. The results of the treatment depend on fracture location (upper, middle, lower third), fracture type (spiral, oblique, transverse), and amount of comminution. The difficulty of treatment is also related to the energy transfer at the time of injury. High-energy fractures are more difficult to heal than low-energy ones. When a car bumper strikes the leg, energy transfer is great in a concentrated zone—this is a high-energy injury. A twisting

FIGURE 24-1

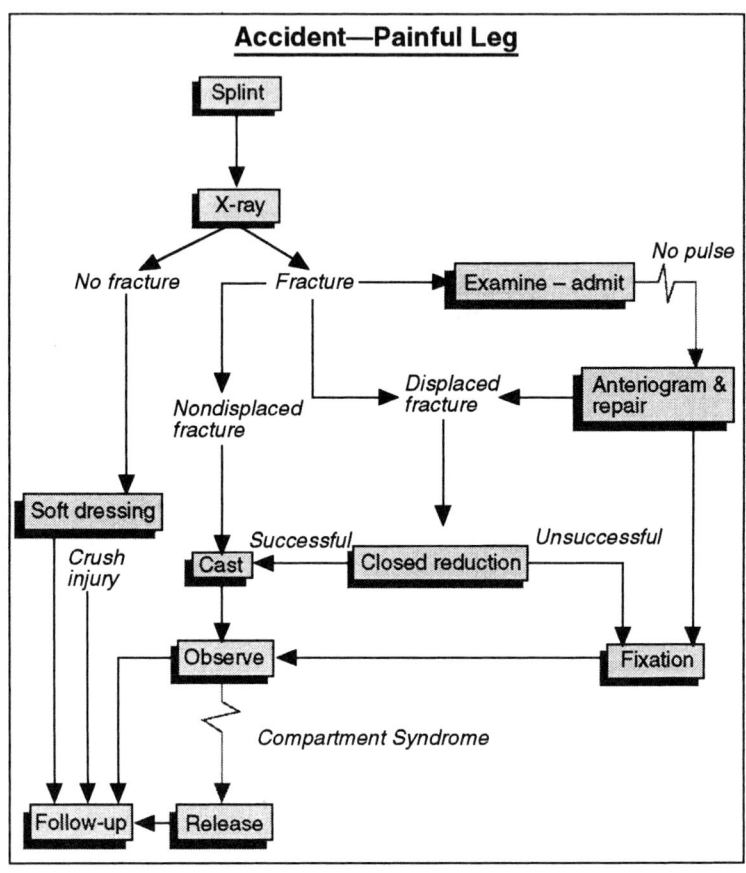

FIGURE 24-1 Accident—painful leg. A patient presenting with leg pain following an accident needs a thorough examination and x-rays (AP and lateral). The exam should include careful evaluation of the skin to rule out open fracture. Neurologic function should be tested and distal pulses palpated. In the event that distal pulses are not palpable, an arteriogram should be obtained to rule out vascular injury. Prior to obtaining x-rays, the involved extremity should be properly splinted to prevent further damage. If x-rays reveal a displaced fracture, closed reduction should be attempted by applying gentle traction. If reduction is successful or if the x-rays reveal a nondisplaced fracture, a bivalved cast should be applied and the patient discharged home to follow up in three to five days. An open fracture, an unsuccessful reduction, or a severely comminuted fracture will require surgical intervention. If a nonbivalved cast is applied, the extremity needs close observation for the development of compartment syndrome. The most sensitive test in the diagnosis of compartment syndrome is pain with passive motion.

fall off a low stool is a low-energy injury. Compounding of the fracture, skin loss, vascular damage, and systemic conditions such as diabetes all delay fracture healing.

After an x-ray, the limb is roughly reduced with gentle traction and placed in a long leg plaster splint. While nonoperative treatment may still be chosen, the precise reduction is usually obtained under anesthesia. Patients with leg fractures are hospitalized to observe for complicating compartment syndromes as the injured limb swells in the first few days following the accident. Healing a leg fracture is a process that takes at least four months.

The operative treatment options include intramedullary nailing (Figure 24-2), bone plating, external fixation, or a combination of methods. Each fracture has a "personality," and treatment is determined by this behavior, as well as by the judgment and experience of the treating physician.

Patients with leg pain and no acute history of trauma may have overuse syndromes, tendinitis, or stress fractures (Figures 24-3, 24-4). Arterial and venous disease needs to be ruled out, particularly in older patients who have leg pain and/or swelling.

FIGURE 24-2 Insertion of an intramedullary nail for an upper femoral fracture. Screws will be placed through the nail into the femoral head (i.e., interlocking screws).

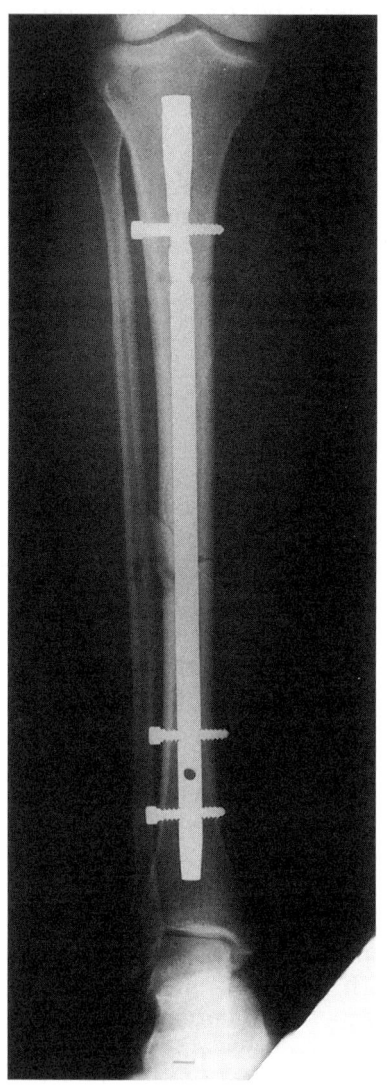

FIGURE 24-3 Spot film of the tibia in a 33-year-old accountant with persistent pain after running a mini-marathon. The film shows nothing.

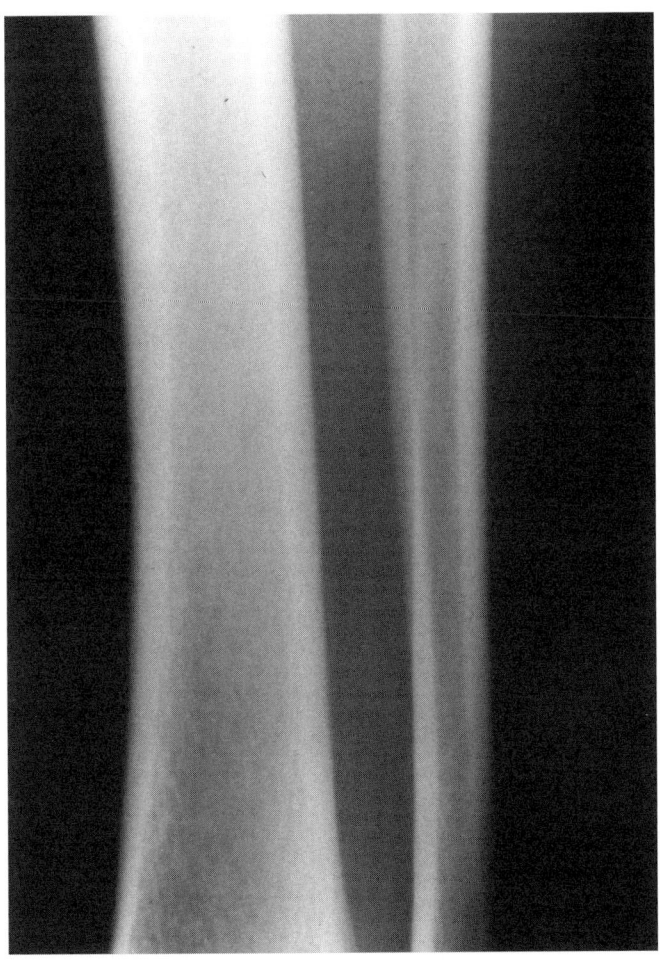

FIGURE 24-4 Bone scan of the same patient one week later shows increased activity in the distal tibia consistent with a stress fracture. The plain x-ray was still negative.

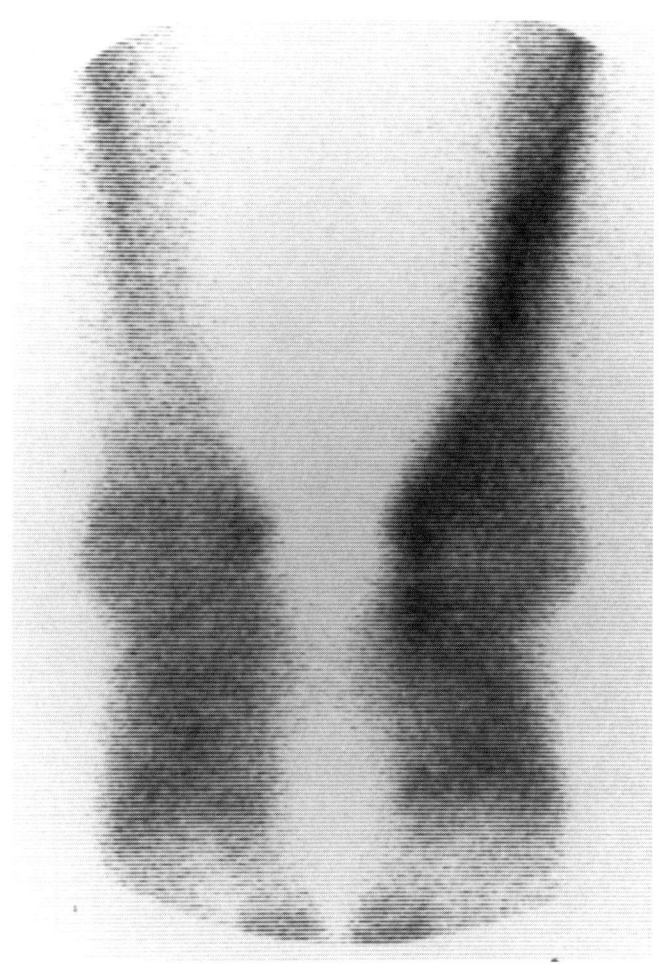

Chapter 25
Ankle Injuries

A. ANKLE SPRAINS

Mild, moderate, severe, and recurrent sprains are common injuries in active young adults. Laterally there are three stabilizing ligaments: the anterotalofibular, the calcaneofibular, and the posterior talofibular ligament (the strongest of the three). The ligament stabilizing the medial aspect of the ankle, the deltoid ligament, consists of five components. The anterior talofibular ligament is the one most often involved in ankle sprains. Ligamentous injuries are graded **type I** for minor injuries, **type II** for incomplete ligamentous injuries, and **type III** for complete ligamentous injuries.

First inspect the ankle for swelling and ecchymosis. Palpate the ankle, noting any tenderness or pain elicited. This localizes the torn ligament. Type III injuries, which involve the complete rupture of the lateral or medial ligaments, are more dramatic than type II injuries, because the magnitude of the injury makes the instability apparent. Sprains of the anterolateral ligaments are diagnosed by local tenderness in the interval between the lateral malleolus and the talus.

In many sprains a telltale bruise develops on the outside of the hindfoot after a few days. Tenderness in the distal interval between tibia and fibula indicates injury to the anterior-inferior tibia-fibula ligament and ankle syndesmosis. On the medial side, the deltoid ligament can be sprained.

To evaluate the lateral ankle ligaments, first place the patient's foot in a plantarflexed and inverted position. If this causes pain, it suggests injury to the ligaments, but does not indicate whether the joint is unstable. Therefore, an anterior drawer test should be performed. An anterior force is applied to the hindfoot and a posteriorly directed force is applied to the distal tibia. A positive test is noted if anterior translation of the talus is detected. This indicates disruption of the calcaneofibular ligament.

Views of the foot and ankle should be obtained to rule out a fracture of the fifth metatarsal and the ankle. If the space between the talus and the tibia, the mortise, is not even all the way around, the ankle injury has a component of significant instability and may need operative repair. Bonnin found an association between the tilt of the talus and degree of ligamentous injury. He found that if there is less than a 15° tilt of the talus, only the anterior talofibular ligament is disrupted. A talar tilt of 15° to 30° indicates that both the anterior talofibular ligament and the calcaneofibular ligaments are disrupted. More than 30° of talar tilt indicates that all three lateral ligaments are torn.

Ankle sprains are immobilized in a splint and reexamined in 2 to 3 days to test for stability. The stable ones can then be treated with an ankle support or ACE bandage, and the unstable ones casted or repaired. Most individuals need crutches after an ankle sprain. An air stirrup is a useful alternative to a splint.

An excessively swollen ankle is occasionally seen that is tender everywhere and this can indicate damage to either the talus or the subtalar joints. Often, however, nothing more than a significant lateral ligament and capsular tear is found. These patients require splinting with plenty of extra padding and need to be off their feet with the leg elevated "toes-above-the-nose" to get them healed as quickly as possible.

B. ANKLE FRACTURES

Ankle fractures and ligamentous injuries are the result of rotational forces acting at the ankle, which produce instability between the tibia and talus. The arch formed by the distal tibia and the fibula is called the ankle **mortise**. The ankle joint has only dorsiflexion and plantar flexion associated with it. Inversion and eversion occur at the subtalar joint, i.e., the joint formed by the talus and calcaneus. In addition to dorsiflexion and plantarflexion, inversion, and eversion, there are four other possible motions at the ankle-foot complex: adduction, abduction, supination, and pronation. Adduction and abduction refer to the forefoot being deviated either medially or laterally, respectively, with respect to the longitudinal axis of the tibia. Supination refers to simultaneous adduction and inversion, while pronation refers to combined abduction and eversion.

Inspect the joint for gross deformity, swelling, or ecchymosis. Assess the neurovascular status. Check dorsalis pedis and posterior tibial pulses. Palpate the joint for focal tenderness medially and laterally, as well as posteriorly.

Take AP, lateral, and internal rotation (mortise) views. Evaluate the AP x-ray for fracture of the medial and lateral malleoli. Also evaluate the lateral view for fracture of the posterior malleolus, and the mortise view for relationships at the distal tib-fib syndesmosis. A torn deltoid ligament has the same functional significance as a fracture of the medial malleolus. The deltoid ligament must be torn or the medial malleolus fractured if the talus lies laterally in the mortise (Figure 25-1).

In the most common fracture pattern the talus rotates outward, splitting apart the distal tibia and fibula, tears the syndesmosis between the two, and fractures the lateral malleolus. Two classification schemes are in use today to categorize ankle fractures: Weber and Lauge-Hansen. The Weber classification is based on the level of the fibula fracture, while Lauge-Hansen is based on the position of the foot and the forces that were acting on it at the time of injury. Only the Weber classification will be described here (see Table 25-1).

Weber type A ankle fractures are usually stable and rarely require ORIF or percutaneously placed cannulated screws. If the fracture in Weber type B is undisplaced, it can be treated with cast immobilization; if displaced, it will need ORIF with placement of a bone plate. Weber C fractures are unstable and need operative repair usually with the placement of a syndesmosis screw from the fibula to the tibia to restore stability to the ankle joint.

FIGURE 25-1 Ankle x-ray. Radiographic evaluation of the ankle requires three views: AP, lateral, and mortise. This figure depicts the mortise view, which is taken with the ankle in 15° of internal rotation and is best suited for visualization of the joint space. The articular surface of the ankle joint should be even all the way around. The cortices of all the involved bones should be examined for irregularities. To rule out ankle instability secondary to ligamentous injury, stress views are necessary.

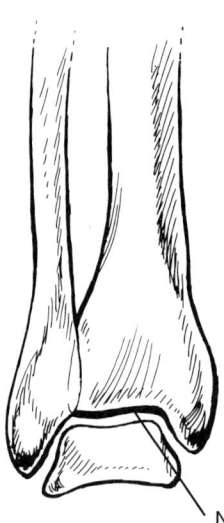

Inspect:
1. Fibula
2. Medial malleolus
3. Fit of talus in the mortise
4. Plafond
5. Talus
6. Calcaneous
7. Base of fifth metatarsal

Note:
The cartilage space must be even all the way around

TABLE 25-1 Weber Classification of Fibula Fractures

TYPE	LEVEL OF FIBULA FRACTURE	PERCENT DISRUPTION OF SYNDESMOSIS
A	Fibula is fractured below the level of the tibial plafond with associated vertical fracture of the medial malleolus.	25%
B	Fibula is fractured at the level of the tibial plafond (usually an oblique fracture) line beginning anteriorly and inferiorly and extending posteriorly and superiorly. The medial malleolus is often avulsed and there also is a posterior lip fracture.	50%
C	The fibula is fractured above the tibial plafond. Also there is a posterior lip fracture, a medial malleolus fracture, or deltoid ligament disruption.	100%

The more proximal the fracture of the fibula and the more components broken, the more unstable the injury (Figure 25-2). *Simple* fractures involving a single malleolus without malposition of the talus in the mortise can be placed in a posterior splint; the patient is given crutches and analgesics and made NWB. Patients need to be instructed to elevate the limb to control swelling. A circular cast is applied a few days later. These injuries can generally be treated in casts or walking orthoses for 6 to 8 weeks.

FIGURE 25-2 In this high-grade (Weber C) fracture of the ankle in a young skier, the talus no longer has the correct relationship to the distal tibia. The medial malleolus is fractured, there is a fracture of the fibula proximal to the joint, and the syndesmotic ligaments are torn.

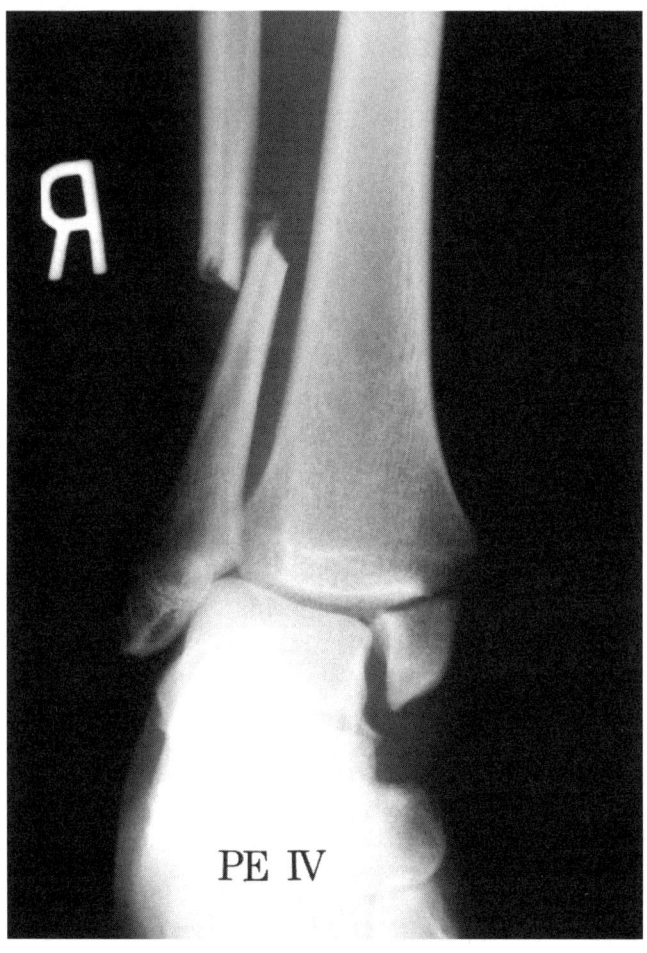

C. PILON FRACTURES

Fractures into the weight-bearing distal tibia articular surface are called pilon fractures. The tibial pilon is also known as the tibial plafond. These fractures are usually caused by axial loading and are often seen in patients who are involved as drivers in motor vehicle accidents and try to prevent injury by pressing hard on the floorboard as the car comes to an abrupt stop (Figure 25-3). Skiers can also sustain this fracture when they come to a stop by skiing into a rock. The severe grades of pilon fractures have compression of the fine cancellous bone of the distal tibia. In these cases, even if the ankle joint surface can be restored, there will be a space that needs to be filled with bone graft.

Once again it is important to assess the vascular status. In addition, careful evaluation of the soft tissue surrounding the joint is imperative, as these fractures are associated with severe swelling and skin problems. Skin slough is not uncommon. Treatment may be further complicated by the presence of an open wound. Also, because of the mechanism of injury, one must look for the presence of spinal and calcaneal compression fractures.

Three views of the ankle—AP, lateral, and ankle mortise views—are taken to identify the injury. In severely injured patients, particularly with open fractures, one view is enough to begin with. Components of the injury can include a fibular fracture (usually a Weber C—see the preceding section), separation of the fibula from the tibia—syndesmosis rupture—and comminution of the central weight-bearing surface of the tibia (i.e., the pilon). The **headset sign** is helpful: the distal tibia sits on the talus like a headpiece on its receiver. When properly seated, the space between the handle and cradle is even—when it is not, injury is present.

Patients need evaluation, well-padded splints, and a careful study of plain x-rays, tomograms, and CT scans to plan their treatment. Unlike malleolus fractures, results of treatment are often imperfect.

The joint surface component can be graded into three grades:

FIGURE 25-3 This patient fractured the distal tibial metaphysis when his car struck a tree. The injury was caused by direct compression of the foot into the floorboard. There is comminution of the metaphysis, extension into the joint, fracture of the fibula, and compression of the bone in the lateral tibia.

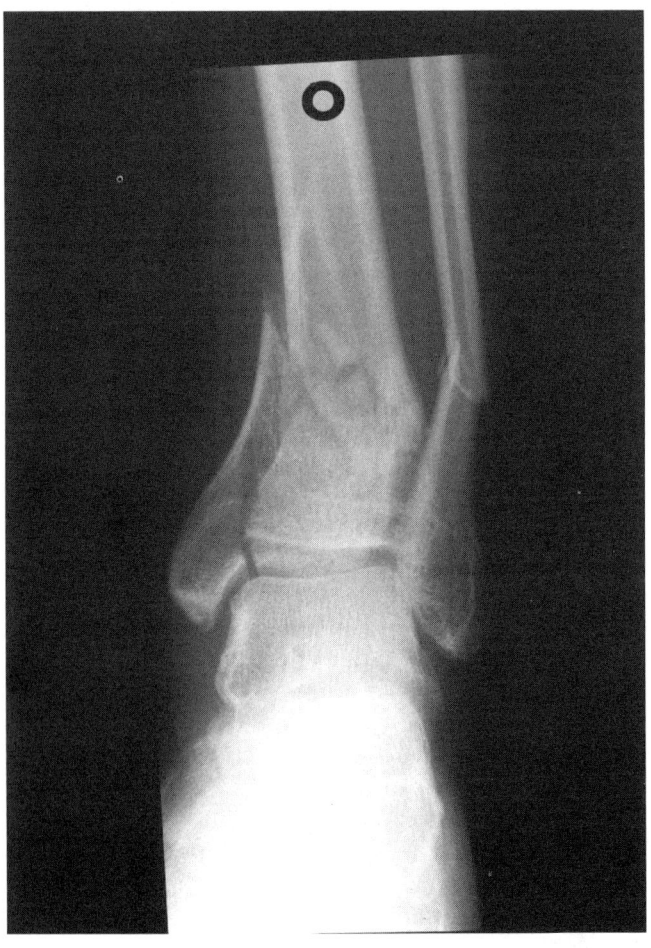

Type A—nondisplaced fractures into the joint
Type B—a few large fragments with joint surface displacement
Type C—severe comminution of the articular surface

Type B and C fractures will require operative reconstruction of the joint surface, often with bone screws.

Open pilon fractures are a dilemma. The best situation is to cover the injury with a sterile saline dressing, take ankle x-rays, and bring the patient promptly to surgery, where a proper debridement can be performed. However, if the patient has multiple injuries and these are life threatening, then the compound pilon fracture is not the first priority. If the skin is tented, in the hours needed for workup of the high-priority injuries the skin will become necrotic. Therefore, despite the risk of folding contaminated material into the wound, it is best to rinse the surface with 200 to 300 cc of sterile saline and reduce the ankle joint with traction on the heel. The key is to inform the trauma team that this was an open dislocation, so an adequate operative treatment can be done when the patient's condition allows.

Since pilon fractures can be caused by abrupt and forceful loading of the ankle, they are often associated with other significant skeletal injuries, so look for spinal and pelvic fractures as well.

Do not underestimate the potential of pilon fractures to cause morbidity. Pilon fractures are associated with severe swelling and skin problems. Skin slough is not uncommon. Patients are at risk for compartment syndrome, fat embolism, and thromboembolism.

As we take thousands of steps each day, the entire weight of the body is concentrated at the tibiotalar joint. Slight degrees of malalignment of the tibia or fibula on the talus and/or residual unevenness of the joint surface set the stage for progressive posttraumatic ankle-joint degeneration. Find the fracture and treat it!

Chapter 26

Foot Fractures

Fractures of the forefoot, midfoot, and hindfoot occur in sports, falls from heights, and automobile accidents.

In the process of walking, as the foot progresses through the gait cycle, its tissues experience pressure (force per unit area) many times greater than body weight. Walking a mile in a half-hour exposes the foot to two thousand cycles. In a day, most people's feet undergo 10,000 cycles—300,000 per month, 3,600,000 a year. Feet are composed of special tissues adapted for this brutal repetitive load.

A foot that has been twisted, bent, landed on from a height, run over by a car, or stomped on by an elephant is not suited for its usual function for at least two to three days postinjury and perhaps longer. Plain x-rays are indispensable for the triage of a foot injury, but they are not good indicators for length of incapacity or type of immediate treatment necessary.

The "history" is one clue to the length of time needed for recovery. A man falling from a roof 20 feet off the ground will take longer to recover than one who fell from a 10-foot scaffolding. Foot injuries cannot be evaluated from x-ray reports. A patient with "normal x-rays" who is told "You have no fractures, so you can work tomorrow," will limp to another emergency room the next morning.

Furthermore, the interpretation of foot x-rays can be difficult because extra bones (sesamoids) and anomalies are frequent. The history, x-ray findings, and location of tenderness must match. A fresh fracture can be distinguished from an old injury or an accessory bone by the normal trabeculation in the fragment, sharp discontinuity at the fracture, and lack of reaction in its edge. Accessory bones and old fragments have sclerotic, radiodense margins.

Another good indicator of the location of injury is the gait pattern. When one walks in normal gait, the heel strikes the floor and one rolls over the foot, finally pushing off from the toes. In midstance, the foot is planted like a tripod with the load distributed equally on the heel and on medial (first metatarsal) and lateral (fifth metatarsal) contact points. If the heel is hurt, the patient walks on the ball of the foot. Conversely, if the forefoot is damaged, the patient makes contact with the heel only and does not roll over the foot. Watch the patient walk over to the stretcher; you can learn a great deal observing the characteristic gait patterns.

Common sports injuries and injuries from everyday activities include toe fractures, metatarsal fractures, and ligamentous avulsions. Major accidents can cause fracture dislocations of the talus and midfoot and calcaneus fractures. Minor fractures are splinted and treated with elevation and analgetics. Major fractures often require hospitalization and operative reduction (see Table 26-1).

All patients need a history of injury and if possible observation of gait. Always compare the injured with the uninjured foot to detect differences in size, shape, color, pulses, and muscle function. Palpate for tenderness. Take plain x-rays.

Provide a no-work statement; use a wrap, soft orthosis, hard-soled shoe, or cast as appropriate for the problem and provide crutches or a cane. Instruct the patient who can go home to elevate the leg "toes above the nose" to control swelling. Prescribe analgetics and arrange for follow-up.

TABLE 26-1 **Common Foot Fractures**

MAJOR	MINOR
Calcaneus	Toes
Talus	Base of fifth metatarsal
Midfoot dislocations	Metatarsal heads

A. FRACTURES AND DISLOCATIONS OF THE TALUS AND CALCANEUS

Since the bones of the hindfoot (talus and calcaneus) are designed for the repetitive high-impact load of walking, fractures of these bones require high energy. These are potentially disabling injuries with uncertain healing. The combination of a typical history, such as a fall from a height or high-speed vehicular trauma, and pain in the heel with difficulty walking suggests hindfoot fracture. Ecchymosis and swelling often do not develop for days after these injuries. Therefore, in polytrauma patients, these fractures may be appreciated only after many days of life-saving care has taken place.

The hindfoot functions like a tripod with the ball of the heel as one leg. Load is carried medially and laterally along the talonavicular and calcaneocuboid axes, respectively. These axes are crossed. The talonavicular axis points toward the great toe, while the calcaneocuboid axis points toward the fifth ray. Identify this relationship on the AP x-ray of the ankle. Then look specifically at the posterior subtalar joint, the talonavicular, and calcaneocuboid joint for fractures. Check the tuberosity of the calcaneus and neck of the talus. In the lateral x-ray, the talus looks like a VW "beetle." Follow the outline of the bone to detect fractures.

Patients with fractures of the talus or calcaneus are placed in a bulky (Jones) dressing and admitted for observation and evaluation. Subsequent swelling and skin blistering are common. Tomography is usually indicated to define the exact fracture anatomy. Operative reduction and bone fixation with screws may be needed. When the talus no longer lies beneath the tibia, an **ankle dislocation** is present. When the calcaneus no longer lies beneath the talus, a **subtalar dislocation** is present. When the talus is dislocated from the tibia and the calcaneus, a **pantalar dislocation** is present. Often with this grave injury there is a fracture of the talar neck, so the talonavicular joint is intact while the rest of the talus is dislocated. These dislocations of the talus from the tibia or of the calcaneus from the talus need to be reduced under anesthesia. Fluoroscopy helps insure that correct relationships have been restored. With fractures through the talar neck, the blood supply to the proximal talus can be lost and bone death (osteonecrosis) follows. Months later, collapse of the talar dome can take place. Many of these patients are never able to return to work that requires standing, climbing, or walking over uneven surfaces. It is thus important to emphasize the gravity of the hindfoot injury from the start of treatment.

B. FOREFOOT FRACTURES AND DISLOCATIONS

Simple closed fractures of the toes and middle metatarsals can be treated as outpatient injuries. Displaced fractures and isolated dislocations are reduced under local infiltration anesthesia. Splint the toe to the adjacent one with tape, and splint the foot in a rocker-bottom cast shoe. The patient will need crutches. Displaced fractures or dislocations of multiple metatarsals may require surgical fixation to restore forefoot balance. Dislocation of the metatarsals from the tarsals, called *Lisfranc's* tarsometatarsal fracture dislocation, is a complex and disabling injury that occurs in several forms. The base of the second metatarsal is keyed into the midfoot and held in place by a ligament to the medial cuneiform. Palpate this area and compare x-rays of both feet. This is an important place to look for injury. Patients with midfoot fractures and dislocations should be admitted for evaluation and careful x-ray assessment.

Fractures of the first and fifth metatarsals prevent weight bearing. The common tendon avulsion of the fifth metatarsal caused by inversion of the foot and avulsion of the peroneous brevis insertion is initially managed non-weight-bearing in a splint. It is not as serious an injury as the diaphyseal cortex-to-cortex fractures of the fifth metatarsal (the Jones fracture), which can take months to unite (Figure 26-1A and B). The Jones' or rebounding fracture occurs when a basketball player comes down hard on the foot. With a bunion the first metatarsal points to the midline (**metatarsus adductus**) and the big toe points lateral (**hallux valgus**). At the apex of this deformity the bunion presents as inflamed soft

FIGURE 26-1 *A.* This basketball player came down on his foot fracturing the fifth metatarsal. The fracture is diaphyseal (the Robert Jones' Fracture).

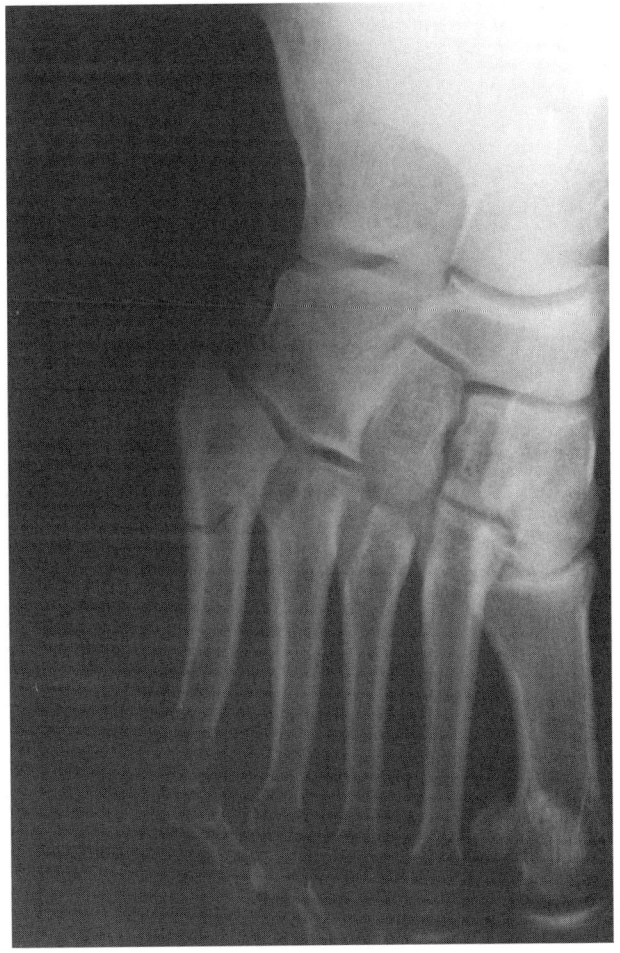

FIGURE 26-1 *(Continued) B.* Several days post-injury it was stabilized with a percutaneous screw in outpatient surgery.

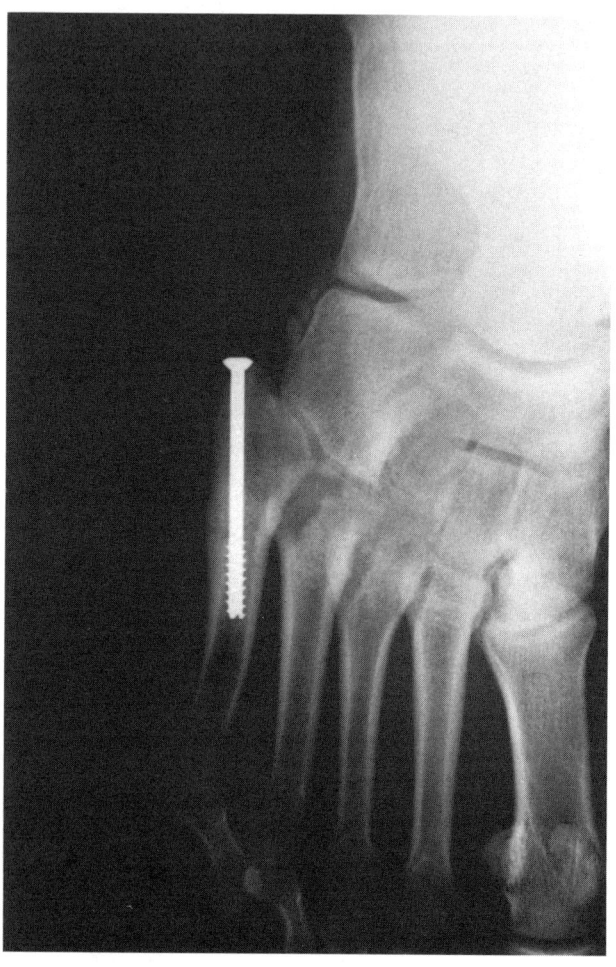

tissue over the metatarsal phalangeal joint (MTP). With gout, the angular deformity is absent. In hallux rigidus there is a ring of painful osteophytes around the MTP joint and diminished motion. Acute foot pain at the first metatarsal phalangeal joint can be caused by a bunion, hallux rigidus, or gout. The heads of the second or third metatarsals are subject to stress fracture and to pressure calluses under the metatarsal heads. Painful pressure calluses can also occur on the dorsum of the toes, particularly when they are deformed. Distinguish between calluses and plantar warts. Warts are often multiple and not related to areas of increased pressure. They have a papillary texture if you scrape a little off the surface with a sterile knife blade.

Patients with painful forefoot conditions should be given a soft dressing, bunion shoe, and a cane or crutches. Initiate antibiotic treatment for infections, suggest foot soaks in warm soapy water, and arrange follow-up with a health provider interested in foot care.

Chapter 27
Spine Fractures

Injury to the spine, be it cervical, thoracic, or lumbosacral, is a justly feared condition. Yet there is a spectrum of presentations, ranging from the unconscious multiple trauma victim strapped to a backboard to the angry ambulatory worker who is doubled up with neck or back pain following a lifting incident. In each situation two pieces of information must be obtained as quickly as possible: the presence of neurologic deficits, and the alignment and structural integrity of the spine. Once these determinations have been made, an appropriate triage can be performed.

It is crucial to identify patients with paralysis from spine fractures, since they can be helped with medication (steroids), decompression, and spine fusion.

The physician who first examines the patient has the best opportunity to observe voluntary movement of all limbs in response to commands. If this information can be reliably obtained before the patient is intubated for an airway problem, then the later care of the severely injured is facilitated. For the present, response to command is the best indicator of function. At some later time, as we have instruments that measure oxygenation (pulse oxygenation), we will have neural monitors. For the moment, the classic neurologic exam—done quickly and recorded accurately—is the gold standard for spine injury.

In the initial neurologic examination, pain, pain upon palpation, and sensory disturbances are not of great diagnostic value. The key is *motor performance*. Ask the patient to move the limbs according to a routine that identifies a level of neurologic deficit. The unconscious patient is harder to evaluate. Intact deep tendon reflexes do not rule out paralysis, they only indicate that the arc is intact. A flaccid patient can have a central cause for lack of reflexes. It is important to record the observation, e.g., "does not withdraw the legs from painful stimuli," and work out the interpretation with the help of specialists in spine trauma.

The most valuable x-ray projection is the lateral view of the spine. In assessing this view, develop the habit of scanning the posterior wall of the vertebral bodies. In any lateral spine view these should be in line, with the posterior wall of each vertebrae lined up with the one above and below on a gentle curve.

Historically, x-rays are ordered and performed according to a protocol based on anatomic region. Thus there are cervical, thoracic, lumbar, and sacral spine exams. Injury is most common, however, at the lower cervical levels or at the thoracolumbar junction. A projection with the beam centered at C5 and at T12 would be better than the standard views of today. Insist that these areas are adequately imaged. A cervical spine film is considered to be inadequate unless the anatomy of the C7 vertebral body is clearly shown.

The negative x-ray and lack of palsy does not rule out disabling soft tissue injury. Do not add to public mistrust of the medical profession by informing the patient that "nothing is wrong." Many patients with these "treated and released" injuries spend months of frustrating interaction with doctors and lawyers until a resolution is reached.

Patients with pain and no acute x-ray changes need a thoughtfully arranged program of medication, soft bracing, "no work" authorization, and early follow-up. Patients with loss of function and fractures need frequent reexamination, documentation of findings, imaging (CT, MRI, myelography), and specialty care. Most other patients who do not have findings on initial examination and plain radiographs will ultimately require added diagnostic tests in the weeks after injury.

In patients with paralysis there are three common clinical patterns:

1. **Transverse myelopathy**—record the lowest level of function

2. **Anterior spinal artery syndrome**—upper extremities are affected more than the lower extremities
3. **Hemisection of the cord**—one leg paralyzed, the other insensate

Then there are phenomena dependent on the state of spinal cord reflexes. When nothing works, the patient is in **spinal shock**—no power on the network. When any one reflex can be found—abdominals, anal wink, bulbocavernosus reflex (elicited by squeezing the glans penis or clitoris and feeling the anus contract)—then power is returning. At this point the neurologic assessment according to Frankel is prognostic (Table 27-1).

Remember that **A** is **A**bsent and **E** is **E**xcellent or normal. In general a patient will advance one Frankel level in recovery. That is, a diver who is paralyzed below C6 (wrist extension) and has no triceps function, but does have abdominal reflexes when examined and can move a toe weakly (useless motor), will probably be able to ambulate when recovered.

Be certain in an emergency assessment not to provide information that you do not have and not to be evasive. Paralysis is terrible and everyone is terrified and angry. Relatives can misinterpret a knee jerk as neurologic function ("But he was moving in the emergency room . . ."). What has been done cannot to this date be undone. More injury must be avoided and communication must not raise false hopes. Kind initial management of an irretrievable situation is a difficult skill to learn.

TABLE 27-1 Frankel's Grades Below a Transverse Lesion

A—No motor function
B—Sensory only
C—Useless motor
D—Useful motor
E—Normal

A. CERVICAL SPINE FRACTURES AND DISLOCATIONS

The triage of neck injuries is a critical area of emergency practice (Figure 27-1). An injury to the cervical spinal cord can cause permanent paralysis. Emergency care is crucial and must be done well. Diagnosis is difficult because the x-rays are hard to interpret. A dislocated neck is easier to miss than a femoral shaft fracture. The way to sort out these cases is to understand the patterns of injury and the associated patient presentations.

There are three basic groups of patients: individuals with paralysis or unconsciousness after an accident; ambulatory patients with neck pain after activity or low-speed injury; and alert patients transported from accidents to the ER in cervical collars. The object is to identify patients with fractures requiring treatment, provided appropriate care and follow-up for those patients with soft tissue damage (whiplash injuries), and safely release the uninjured from cervical immobilization. Every conscious patient should first have a quick survey of the motor function of the lower cervical levels. Use Table 27-2.

Patients who have weakness, report sensory change, or are unconscious have a fractured cervical spine until proven otherwise. They are x-rayed in immobilization, and if necessary for diagnosis they are admitted, films are reviewed, and special studies are obtained. Cervical spine injuries should be treated thoughtfully—never hastily. Unlike bleeding or airway problems, they do not demand speed. Work slowly and accurately. To *save* neurologic function, as in saving for retirement, think **IRA**. *Immobilize* first, then *Radiograph,* and finally *Assess* the problem.

Immobilization is accomplished on a long or short backboard. Most patients will come to the emergency room in the device. Both the head and torso must be secured. The patient who is fastened by the head alone is in real danger if the body is rotated. Immobilization must be maintained until the cervical spine films are reviewed and "cleared."

The sequence for x-ray evaluation of the unconscious or neurologically compromised patient is to first take a scout lateral x-ray in immobilization. If no fracture or dislocation is

FIGURE 27-1 Suspected neck injury. In the patient with a suspected cervical spine injury, it is imperative that the C-spine be immobilized in a rigid collar. Assess the patient's neurologic function. Record the results and the time of the exam, because in the course of serial examinations it will be necessary to ascertain whether the patient's neurologic status is deteriorating and at what rate. If there is a sensory deficit, determine the sensory level as it corresponds to dermatome distribution. Obtain C-spine films, the most important of which is the lateral view. Ensure that the film is adequate by being able to visualize the C7–T1 disc space. If the patient experiences tenderness to palpation, and x-rays show no evidence of fracture or dislocation, then flexion/extension views should be obtained. If these are negative, the patient can be placed in a soft collar and released with analgesics to follow up in three to five days. In the case of neurologic deficit and an unstable injury pattern, further radiographic imaging needs to be performed. Unstable injuries will require placement of tongs or halo-vest with or without surgical repair.

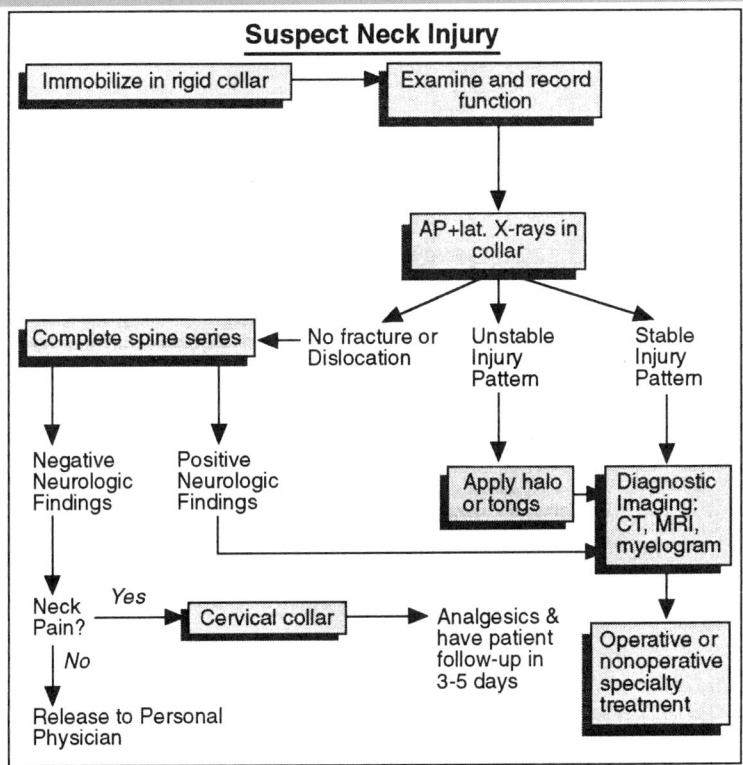

TABLE 27-2 Quick Assessment of Motor Function of Conscious Patient

LEVEL	MUSCLE	QUESTION
C5	Biceps	Bend your elbow
C6	Extensor carpi radialis	Bring up your wrist
C7	Triceps	Straighten your elbow
C8	Forearm flexors	Squeeze my hand

present, the backboard or collar is removed and a full series is taken, which shows at least the superior surface of the first thoracic vertebra.

The forces, such as diving into a pool and striking one's head, that cause fracture and/or paralysis are much greater than those that occur during care of the patient in a medical facility. A rigid collar or sandbags will suffice to prevent additional injury. Gentle traction with the neck in slight extension is the safest position for transfers, since most injury vectors involve flexion and compression. The protection against spinal motion provided by the common appliances is least with a soft collar and greatest with a halo cast. Rigid braces are intermediate (see Table 27-3).

TABLE 27-3 Cervical Spine Immobilization

PROTECTION	DEVICE
Least	Soft cervical collar
Intermediate	Sandbags
	Hard Philadelphia collar
	SOMI (sternal occipital Mandibular immobilizer)
Most	Tongs—traction
	Halo—vest
	Halo—cast

Neurologically intact patients, though they may not report neck pain, must have cervical spine x-rays taken to complete their evaluation, but those films can be obtained out of the collar. Pain does not rule in or rule out neck injury. It is one finding that can be factored into the decision-making process. Face and scalp bruises and lacerations are another clue to the presentation of a cervical spine injury.

When the x-rays show an **unstable** spine or when the patient has paralysis, the next step is for a specialist to place the patient in skeletal traction with either tongs or a halo. Unstable spines have either dislocation, multiple fractures, or significant angulation (Figure 27-2). Stable fractures are minor compressions, lower-level (C5 to C7) spinous process fractures, and anterior vertebral body avulsion fractures.

Many older patients have marked degenerative changes in the cervical spine (cervical spondylosis). Their x-rays are really uninterpretable. Here, if the neurological exam is negative and they are mobile but have pain, use a soft cervical collar and arrange for prompt follow-up. A bone scan, tomogram, or flexion-extension x-rays may be needed for diagnosis, and this may take some time. Most will require therapy, medication, and time off work.

Set the stage from the beginning of medical care for compassionate care of the patient with "negative" x-rays. Significant soft tissue injury may be present. The relationship of a plain x-ray to the conditions of the neck is like comparing a wallet-sized black-and-white photo to a technicolor movie. Pain without paralysis arises in discs, facet joints, muscles, and ligaments. It may become worse hours or days after the injury as the patient tries to resume activity. These patients become concerned, confused, and frightened. They have more pain from muscle spasms and nowhere to go. Appointments may be hard to schedule. Sophisticated diagnostic imaging may be expensive and not provide answers.

Take a moment to explain the injury, provide adequate pain medication, and arrange prompt follow-up. Remember that the patient will come in contact with well-meaning people who want answers. These include friends, relatives, insurance agents, police, and even lawyers. The patient with pain and no answers fares poorly when advised not to work until

FIGURE 27-2 This 22-year-old college student dove into a swimming pool and hit his head. He had transient numbness and paralysis of the legs. The lateral x-ray of the cervical spine shows widening between the spinous processes of C4 and C5, separation of the facets, and angulation between the vertebral bodies. This is an unstable situation.

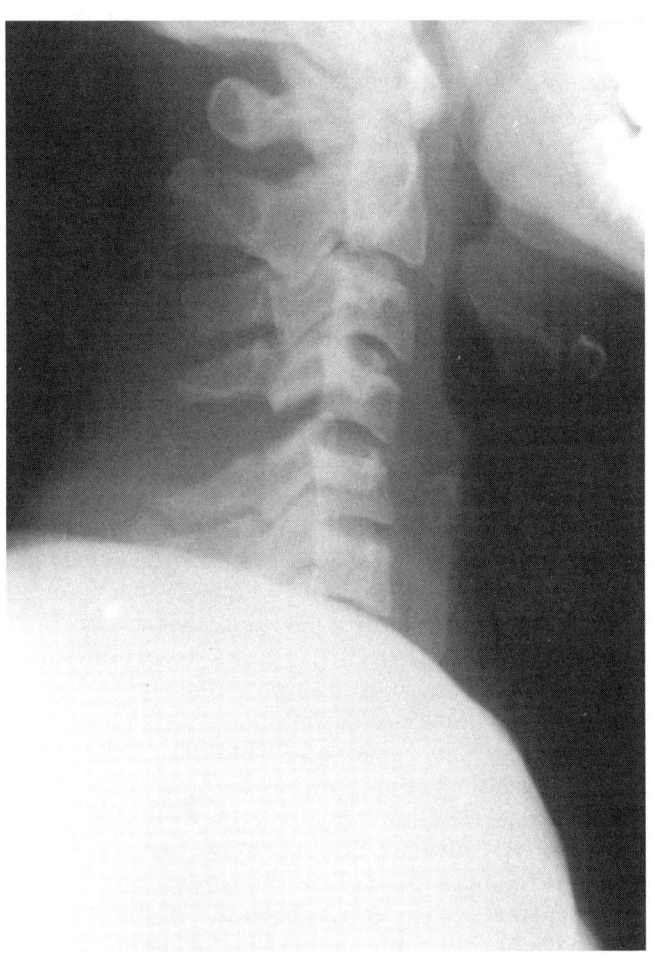

"pain free." Then bills and responsibilities accumulate and a vicious cycle of disability, depression, and discouragement begins. The emergency room is the place to practice preventive medical education by acknowledging that the patient has injury even though there may be no neurologic damage and the x-rays are "normal" (Figure 27-3).

B. THORACOLUMBAR FRACTURES

Significant fractures and fracture dislocations of the thoracolumbar spine are the product of high-speed and significant trauma. Unconscious patients with thoracolumbar spine fractures or patients with neurologic findings in the legs require exacting care. Meticulous documentation of the physical examination, early administration of high-dose corticosteroids, and thoughtful organization of the diagnostic workup and specialty planning for a possible operative approach are mandatory. The examination of the completely paralyzed patient for primitive cord reflexes (abdominals, cremasteric, bulbocavernosus) is the same as for neck injuries. The knee and ankle jerks are recorded as present, increased, diminished, or absent. Plantar responses are upward or downward. The time it takes to write out the details in legible language or to prepare unambiguous charts is well spent.

Injuries caused by lifting, simple falls, and stooping or twisting either sprain the supporting intervertebral ligaments, damage lower lumbar discs, or—in the elderly or other patients with osteoporosis—compress thoracic or lumbar vertebrae. Compression fractures and lumbar sprains cause pain and muscle spasm seemingly out of proportion to the radiographic findings. If the patient can actively "set" the knee and dorsiflex the foot or great toe and plantarflex the foot against resistance, significant neurological damage is unlikely. Nonetheless, patients with these stable injuries benefit from sympathetic treatment, which may include short-term hospitalization for pain control and rehabilitation under supervision.

In awake patients, spot-check the neural axis from the quadriceps **(L3),** foot dorsiflexors **(L4),** great toe extensors

FIGURE 27-3 The lateral cervical spine x-ray. Evaluation of the lateral C-spine must begin with determining whether the film is adequate. In order for the study to be adequate, all seven cervical vertebral bodies must be visualized. Prior to examination of the bony elements, evaluate the surrounding soft tissues. Acceptable limits for soft tissue are 7 mm at C2, 22 mm at C6, and 3 mm from the atlas to the dens. Measurements greater than these limits may indicate edema or hematoma and should be evaluated further. A line drawn down the posterior border of the vertebral bodies should be smooth and uninterrupted. A line that is interrupted indicates trauma or a degenerative process. Examine each vertebral body for size and shape. A decrease in the size of the vertebral body may indicate a burst or compression fracture.

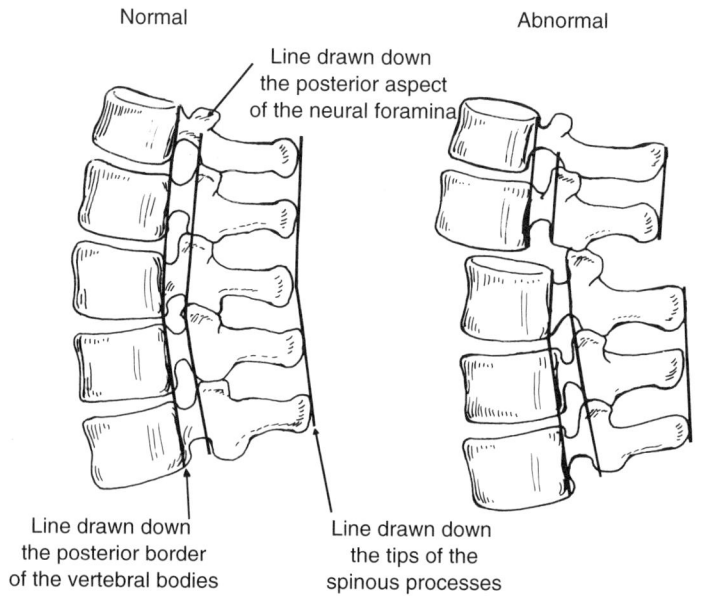

(**L5**) to the plantar flexors (**S1**). ("Lumbar *three* runs over the *knee*.") Motor findings are generally more useful than the sensory exam, but do note diminished sensation on the side opposite a motor deficit. Keep the patient on a backboard and use a team of at least three to turn the patient "**en bloc**" to examine the posterior surface or to change sheets or remove clothing until a spine specialist has had the opportunity to review the physical findings and the x-rays and plan further care.

Basic x-rays are taken on large plates. The AP hips and pelvis and flat plate of the chest and abdomen combined with a "shoot through" lateral centered at the thoracolumbar junction are a good scout series for the common major fracures and dislocations. Be warned that the lateral chest may not show upper thoracic fractures clearly. If the arms are in the way, move them and shoot again. A CT scan or lateral linear tomogram may be the only way to clear the upper thoracic spine (C7–T8).

Remembering that x-rays are like snapshots, i.e., they do not reveal what happens when the spine moves. There can be ligamentous disruption without fracture, and this disruption can paralyze. The basic injury patterns are compression, burst fracture with neural compromise secondary to fragments of vertebral body propulsed into the spinal canal, slice fractures across the vertebral body from a shear force, and flexion or extension fracture-dislocation.

One useful concept is to divide the spine into "columns": (1) an anterior column with vertebral body and anterior and posterior longitudinal ligaments, and (2) posterior columns with pedicles and facet joints, laminae, spinous processes, and interspinous ligaments. Injury to both of these columns means instability.

In general when there is marked angulation to one side (scoliosis) or angulation with a posterior apex (kyphosis) or bone in the spinal canal or fractures in a vertebral body and its posterior elements (fracture front and back), then operative decompression and fusion will be necessary.

In triage, at the least, patients with thoracolumbar fractures from major trauma are put in the hospital for observation. They need an IV, baseline labs (Hct, Hgb, WBC,

PT/PTT, and urinalysis), and sequential observation of neurologic function.

Any loss of function under observation requires immediate action. Find the specialist responsible for care and organize subsequent steps in diagnosis and treatment. Imaging (MRI, CT, myelogram) or surgery (decompression-fusion) may be indicated.

It is important at least for the first 24 hours to keep spine-injured patients NPO—not only because they may require urgent intervention, but also because many of them develop paralytic ileus as a consequence of their spinal injury. A nasogastric tube is usually indicated. Unconscious or severely injured patients need a urinary catheter. Repeat the laboratory screen after 12 hours—trends are always more informative than single data points.

Elderly patients with osteoporosis or patients with diminished bone mass, caused, for example, by corticosteroids or renal failure, can sustain thoracolumbar vertebral body fractures from minor trauma—even sitting down hard in an unexpectedly low chair or picking up a grandchild. These fractures are intensely painful. On the lateral x-ray compare the heights of the posterior wall of the thoracic or lumbar vertebra. They get larger at each successive level. Vertebral body size should be in order. Often patients have multiple fractures of varying age. Gently tap on the spinal processess with a reflex hammer. Sharp pain at a spinal level is a sign of acute fracture (**Palmer's test**). These patients can be fearful of falling apart. Their fears are not unjustified. Compression fractures are not usually associated with neural compromise and can be treated with supportive bracing like a soft lumbosacral support. In the months after compression fracture additional settling occurs. Small compression fractures in osteoporotic bone can be treated without hospitalization, but follow-up should be arranged for a few days after injury.

C. ACUTE LOW BACK PAIN

Injuries caused by lifting, twisting, stooping, simple falls, and low-speed collisions cause back pain. Patients with prior lumbar spine surgery have recurrent back pain. And sometimes there is no clear event that precipitates a painful back.

Patients present to the ER, sometimes under their own power and sometimes by ambulance, seeking answers on occasion to problems they have had for years, accompanied by multiple medications, numerous special studies including MRI, CT, and myelogram, and defensive pain- and fear-directed behavior. We do poorly. We would rather cardiovert a heart, push bicarbonate, or place a chest tube than listen to a fellow traveler with a sore back.

The first thing to do is to find out what actually hurts. The patient may sign in with "back pain" and you may even have a set of lumbar films and be thinking "low back pain" when what they mean is pain between the shoulder blades. Ask the patient to make a sketch on a blank piece of paper and mark all the painful areas. They can do this if they must wait, and the sketch can be helpful in diagnosis.

Discogenic back pain waxes and wanes. This is thought due to the changing state of hydration of the intervertebral disc. Back pain is relieved lying down: intradiscal pressure is less. Coughing increases the pain because coughing increases intradiscal pressure.

Findings are divided into mechanical consequences of low back injury and neurologic problems. For every hundred patients with a sore low back there will be less than one with a "pinched nerve" caused by a herniated disc.

If the patient can actively "set" the knee and dorsiflex the foot or great toe and plantarflex the foot against resistance, significant neurological damage is unlikely.

Those patients with new onset weakness and positive sciatic stretch tests will need a detailed workup in a specialty outpatient setting. It is only a rare case where an acute massive central disc rupture causing paralysis presents emergently, and then admission is required.

The mechanical signs of disc injury include restricted motion, crooked back (**sciatic scoliosis**), tight lower lumbar muscles, and hamstring tightness on straight leg raising.

The neurologic findings of pinched nerve can be divided into nerve *conduction* and nerve root *irritation* abnormalities.

Conduction abnormalities are weakness, sensory loss, and reflex changes. Since the L5 and S1 nerve roots are the most commonly affected levels, strength in dorsiflexion of the great toe (L5) and the Achilles' reflex (S1) are the two best tests for conduction abnormality.

Nerve root irritation can be an acute finding. Irritation is also common in patients after disc surgery. Burning, vague pain in the posterior thighs or aching in the heel are findings of nerve root irritation.

The work-up for low back pain includes history, examination for mechanical and neurologic findings, and a set of lumbar films including at least an AP, lateral, and spot film of the lumbosacral junction. Most of the low back pain problems are a result of damage to a disc and its supportive structures. X-ray findings include disc space narrowing, osteophyte formation, and facet joint arthritis. Translation of a lumbar vertebral body anteriorly (**spondylolithesis**) can occur on a degenerative basis. Note that the x-ray findings reflect the entire mechanical history of the patient's back. Therefore, the structure producing pain may not be the one observed on the x-ray.

Several distinct clinical entities apart from pure lumbar disc disease should be kept in mind; these include lumbosacral spondylolithesis, spinal stenosis, and disc space infection (Table 27-4).

Back-pain patients can be sent home from the ER, but after a good workup they need some answers. Most need a time-limited "no-work" statement (five days is usually enough). They

TABLE 27-4 Some Lumbar Spine Conditions

CONDITION	POPULATION	PATHOLOGIC SIGNS
Spondylolithesis	Young adults	Hamstring spasm
Disc space infection	All ages	Terrible pain even lying down
Spinal stenosis	Elderly	Neurogenic claudication

need a place for follow-up: the appointment should be definite. Short-term medication that alleviates pain must be prescribed. Physical measures such as crutches, lumbar support, and suggestions for position in bed are also helpful. Strict bed rest is no longer the gold standard of nonoperative care for disc problems. Patients should be advised against activities that aggrevate discogenic pain, such as sitting for prolonged periods or operating heavy equipment.

PART III

CASE HISTORIES AND SELF-TEST

Case A

L. S., a four-year-old boy, fell off a couch. He landed on his left hand and had the onset of pain and deformity. His parents brought him to the emergency department, where an x-ray was taken (Figure A-1).

1. ***L. S. sustained***
   - **a)** displaced metaphyseal fractures of the distal radius and ulna.
   - **b)** "greenstick" fractures of the distal radius and ulna.
   - **c)** comminuted fractures of the radius and ulna with an elbow dislocation.
   - **d)** articular fracture of the radius and ulna with radial head dislocation.
   - **e)** torus fractures of the radius and ulna.

2. ***This fracture most likely***
   - **a)** will be treated in a splint on an outpatient basis.
   - **b)** will require open reduction and internal fixation.
   - **c)** will need some form of anesthesia in order to achieve an acceptable reduction.
   - **d)** should be managed in external fixation.
   - **e)** is frequently associated with neurovascular compromise.

3. ***The history of injury is suspicious. A referral to the appropriate agency for suspected child abuse (trauma X) is***
   - **a)** inappropriate: the fracture type is not typical for trauma X.
   - **b)** not appropriate unless other injuries are evident.
   - **c)** appropriate: fracture of both bones of the forearm is "classic" for trauma X.
   - **d)** a waste of time.

FIGURE A-1 Injury x-ray in Case A.

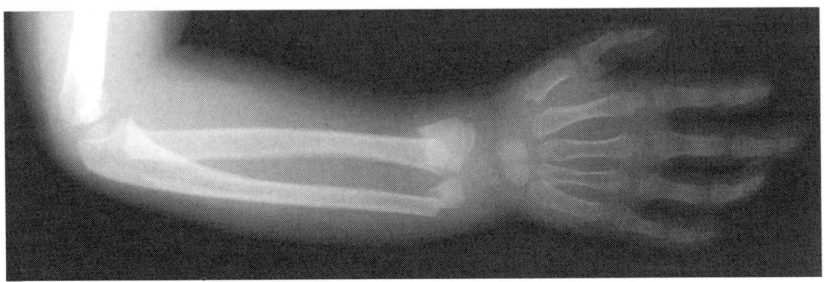

4. *Signs and symptoms of ischemia from a tight cast that can lead to permanent muscle damage are*
   a) pain in the forearm.
   b) swelling and paralysis of the fingers.
   c) pain on passive stretch of the fingers.
   d) loss of sensation of the hand.
   e) some or all of the above.

Answers: 1. a), 2. c), 3. b), 4. e).

Discussion:

Transverse fractures of the distal metaphysis of the forearm are the pediatric equivalent of "Colles" nonarticular fracture of the distal radial metaphysis with dislocation of the distal ulna in adults. Manipulative reduction is much easier under anesthesia. Sometimes a "pediatric cocktail" is sufficient. The fractures can be splinted if the patient is to be sent home. Probably a circular cast that is split and overnight observation (23-hour) is the safest plan. Definitive treatment will be in a circular cast. The position needs to be checked by x-ray in 7 to 10 days as the fracture is becoming sticky. Four weeks of immobilization is sufficient. Trauma X fractures are usually multiple and often spiral torsion injuries. However, any fracture pattern can be present. The tip-off is the presence of many injuries in different stages of healing.

Case B

D. T., a 24-year-old company sales representative, returned from jogging and drove his car back along the route to check the mileage. He ran into a tree, fractured his left wrist on the steering wheel, and broke his right femur (Figure B-1) when his knee struck the dash. Fortunately, the air bag inflated, and he sustained no internal injuries. There was no loss of consciousness. He was brought to the hospital with a traction splint on his right leg, a backboard, and a cervical collar.

1. *Which of the following statements concerning the patient's treatment is true?*
    a) The traction splint should be removed, the leg inspected, and x-rays taken.
    b) The leg should be left in traction and x-rays taken in the splint.
    c) Maintain traction, remove clothing, replace the splint, and take x-rays.
    d) X-rays of the femur are of low priority; they can be taken at the time of surgery.
    e) A single x-ray of the femur shaft is all that will be needed to plan care.

2. *The initial workup on the patient should include which of the following?*
    a) Hct, WBC, urine, electrolytes, prothrombin time, type and crossmatch 2 units.
    b) Hct, WBC, urine, and electrolytes.
    c) Hct, WBC, urine, type and screen.
    d) Hct, prothrombin time, urine, and electrolytes.
    e) The initial lab should be as economical as possible.

3. *It will be useful to have which of the following?*
    a) Butterfly IV, nasogastric tube, and a Doppler monitor of the pedal pulse.

186 CASE HISTORIES AND SELF-TEST

FIGURE B-1 Injury x-ray in Case B.

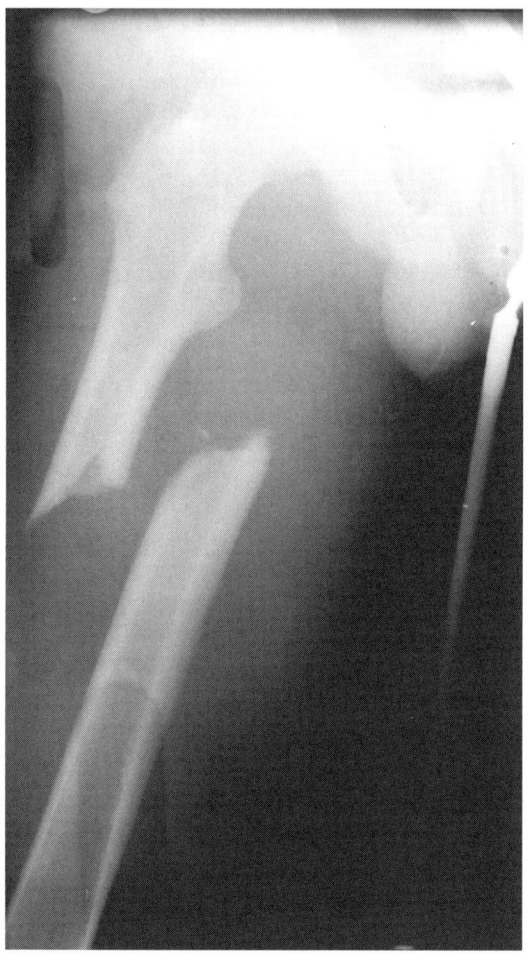

b) Arterial line, cardiac monitor, and a Foley catheter.
c) Swan-Ganz catheter, cardiac monitor, Foley catheter, and oxygen by nasal prongs.
d) Central venous line, Foley catheter, nasogastric tube, and a cardiac moniter.
e) Adequate IV access, Foley catheter, nasogastric tube, and oxygen by nasal prongs.

4. *This fracture is best described as*
a) open butterfly.
b) comminuted transverse.
c) simple oblique.
d) transverse midshaft.
e) complex comminuted.

Answers: 1. c), 2. a), 3. e), 4. c).

Discussion:

Fractures of the femur shaft are managed by intramedullary nailing. Nonsurgical options are less frequently used. The initial workup is directed at finding occult injuries. It is important to have adequate femur x-rays to show the bone from hip to knee. A nondisplaced femoral neck fracture can be present. Intoxicated patients or patients with head injury require more screening. The fractured limb should be handled in traction to avoid additional muscle damage from the broken bone ends and to facilitate surgery by maintaining length. Significant blood loss accompanies the injury and subsequent surgery. Supplemental oxygen is a prophylaxis against fat embolism syndrome.

Case C

M. J. C., a 25-year-old woman, was at her bachelorette party. She was outside barefoot, looking over the fence trying to catch a glimpse of her fiancé. Her friends sent her back in for some shoes. She put on some flats and returned to the fence. As she was straining over to have a good look, she slipped, fell and hurt her foot. She came to the emergency department and an x-ray was taken (Figure C-1). Her main concern was being able to walk down the aisle at her wedding, which was planned for the week after the injury.

1. **On physical examination there is pain and ecchymosis along the hindfoot. The x-ray (Figure C-1) shows**
   a) nothing: the patient has had an ankle sprain.
   b) fracture of the base of the fifth metatarsal at the insertion of the peroneus brevis tendon.
   c) an accessory bone (sesmoid) at the base of the fifth metatarsal.
   d) a Robert-Jones fracture of the fifth metatarsal.
   e) a middle phalanx fracture of the fourth toe.

2. **The treatment for this injury**
   a) will require outpatient surgery to replace the bone fragment with the tendon insertion.
   b) will necessitate hospitalization, repair and immobilization in a cast.
   c) can be accomplished with a splint or soft dressing, but she will be unable to walk down the aisle.
   d) can be accomplished so she can be weight bearing and walk down the aisle.
   e) cannot be planned until additional studies including a CT of the foot are obtained.

FIGURE C-1 Injury x-ray in Case C.

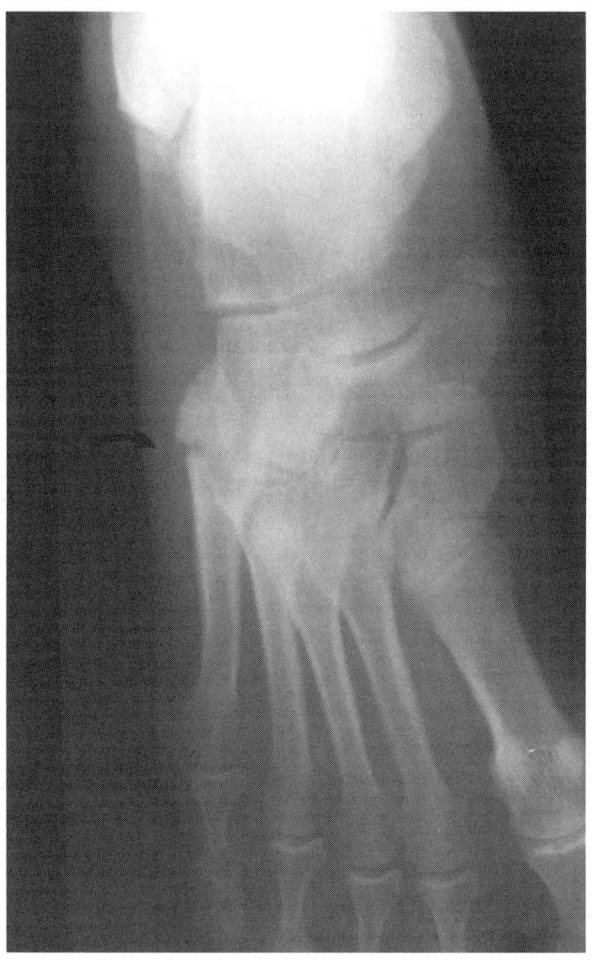

3. **M. J. C. is treated in the emergency department and released. Her care should include**
   a) a short leg splint, crutches, and analgesics.
   b) written instructions on cast care.
   c) a follow-up appointment within 2 to 5 days.
   d) (a), (b), and (c).
   e) just (c); (a) increases cost and (b) is unnecessary.

4. *The splint for this injury*
   a) extends from the toes to the malleoli with the foot plantar flexed.
   b) extends from the metatarsal heads to the proximal calf with the foot at a right angle to the leg (plantigrade).
   c) extends along the lateral border of the foot.
   d) extends from the toes to the malleoli with the foot dorsiflexed.
   e) places the foot in eversion to relax peroneous brevis.

Answers: 1. b), 2. d), 3. d), 4. b).

Discussion:

Avulsion-fracture at the base of the fifth metatarsal is common and also commonly overlooked. Since the area of maximum tenderness is close to the talar insertion of the anterior talofibular ligament, it can be confused with a sprain of the lateral ligaments of the ankle. The injury causes swelling, local pain, and ecchymosis along the lateral border of the heel. Ankle x-rays frequently omit this area or show it imperfectly. It is better to order "foot and ankle" films to rule out this injury. After a few days of splinting and non-weight bearing this fracture can be treated with tape or an elastic bandage (e.g., ACE). Active patients are sometimes more comfortable in a walking short leg cast. The initial splint should be made with the foot plantigrade—at right angles to the tibia. If this is not done, it can be difficult to get the foot flat even after only a few days because of a heel cord contracture. A short leg splint should always extend from the high calf to the metatarsal heads or out to support the toes, so that if the patient falls, the tibia does not fracture on the splint. Healing may be by fibrous union, but the functional result of nonoperative treatment is good (Figure C-2).

FIGURE C-2 Healing fracture at 3 months in Case C.

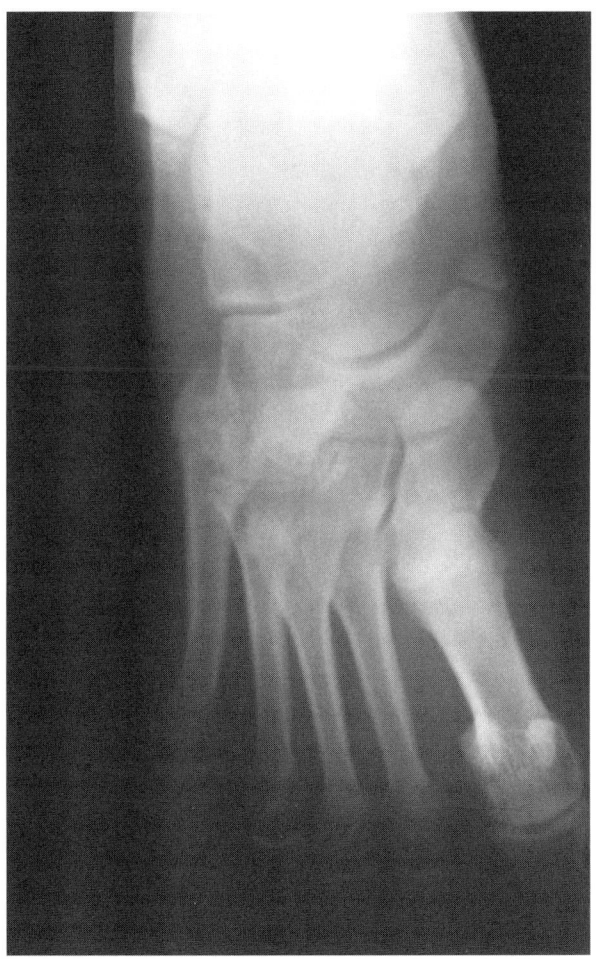

Case D

M. B., a 50-year-old woman interior painter and wallpaper hanger, fell from a ladder, landing on her buttocks. She had the immediate onset of intense back pain and tingling in her legs. She was transported on a backboard by EMS to the emergency department. Initial physical examination revealed that major motor groups of the lower limbs were intact. An x-ray was taken (Figure D-1).

Match the motor function in column A with the nerve root in column B.

	A	B
1.	_____ Hip flexors	a) $L_{2,3}$
2.	_____ Hip extensors	b) $L_{3,4}$
3.	_____ Knee extensors	c) $L_{4,5}$
4.	_____ Knee flexors	d) L_5, S_1
5.	_____ Foot dorsiflexors	e) $S_{1,2}$
6.	_____ Foot plantar flexors	

7. *The injury is described as*
   a) a slice fracture.
   b) a burst injury.
   c) a wedge compression fracture.
   d) a teardrop extension fracture.
   e) a teardrop flexion fracture.

8. *This may be an unstable injury, therefore*
   a) the patient can be moved to a regular bed.
   b) the patient can be moved to a Stryker frame.
   c) the patient can be placed in a wheelchair.
   d) the patient can get up and walk.
   e) more information (e.g., C.T., M.R.I., or lateral tomograms is required.

FIGURE D-1

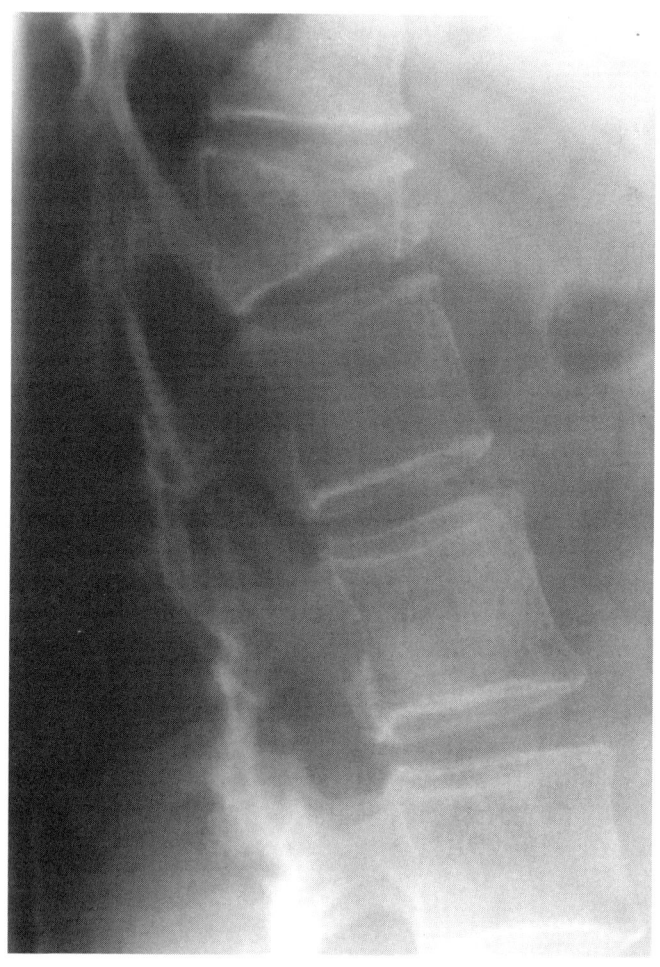

9. *The appropriate ER treatment should include*
   a) an IV.
   b) a Foley catheter.
   c) a nasogastric tube.
   d) (a) and (c).
   e) (a), (b), and (c).

Answers: 1.a), 2. c), 3. b), 4. d), 5. c), 6. e), 7. c), 8. e), 9. d).

Discussion:

Stability and instability are relative terms. If, under treatment, displacement occurs with possible neurologic damage, the fracture was unstable. As a general rule, when there is damage to the spine anteriorly (vertebral body, ligaments) and posteriorly (pedicles, laminae, facets), the fracture is unstable. Wedge compression fractures are usually stable. However, the history of transient sensory disturbance is a caution. Ileus is not uncommon, and overnight nasogastric suction prevents uncomfortable gastric distention. If the patient can void, a Foley catheter is not necessary. Progressive spinal deformity (kyphus) with pain and long tract signs can occur, but most of these injuries can be treated by bracing.

Case E

M. P., a 20-year-old college basketball player, jumped up to rebound, raised his right hand, was hit from behind, and came down with intense right shoulder pain. There was a loss of fullness to inspection of the right shoulder and an area of numbness over the lateral aspect of the arm. He was taken by the trainer to the emergency department where a shoulder x-ray was taken (Figure E-1).

1. *The x-ray shows*
    a) a clavicle fracture.
    b) an acromion fracture.
    c) a shoulder dislocation, probably anterior.
    d) a shoulder dislocation, probably posterior.
    e) a coracoid process fracture.

2. *Reduction*
    a) can probably be accomplished in the ER with a gentle closed technique.
    b) will require a general anesthetic, because this is a first dislocation in a heavily muscled athlete.
    c) is hazardous, because there are signs of nerve damage.
    d) carries a significant risk of fracture of the upper humerus.
    e) will be easy, because this is a first dislocation in an athlete.

Match the motor function in column A with the peripheral nerve in column B

	A	B
3. ____	elbow flexion	a) median nerve
4. ____	wrist extension	b) radial nerve
5. ____	thumb flexion	c) ulnar nerve
6. ____	little-finger adduction	d) musculocutaneous

FIGURE E-1 Injury x-ray in Case E.

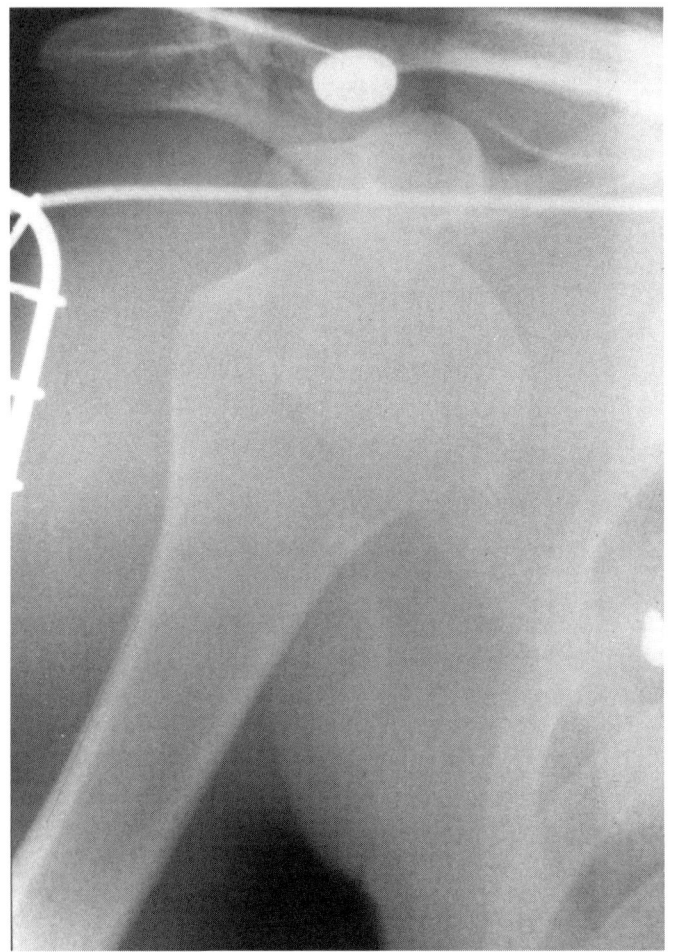

7. *Following reduction an x-ray was taken (Figure E-2). The patient*
   a) will be admitted for overnight observation of neurologic function.
   b) will be admitted for open or arthroscopic reconstruction of the shoulder capsule.
   c) will be placed in a plaster velpeau immobilizer and sent home.
   d) will be placed in a cradle arm sling and sent home.
   e) will be placed in a sling and strap or swathe to prevent external rotation and sent home.

Answers: 1. c), 2. a), 3. d), 4. b), 5. a), 6. c), 7. e).

Discussion:

Shoulder dislocation is a painful injury. Age less than 30 and absence of a greater tuberosity fracture are poor prognostic signs for recurrence. Most active young adults will develop symptoms of anterior instability—a feeling of laxity in the joint—or redislocation. They will ultimately undergo open or arthroscopic reconstruction of the torn shoulder capsule, depending on the extent of the bone and soft tissue injury. Most dislocations are anterior, but a second x-ray projection (transthoracic or scapular view) is necessary to be sure. Axillary nerve palsy manifested by numbness of the lateral arm is a common finding that usually resolves. The arm should be placed in internal rotation for three weeks (i.e., with a sling and swathe or a sling and strap) to give the best chance for a stable shoulder.

FIGURE E-2 Postreduction x-ray in Case E.

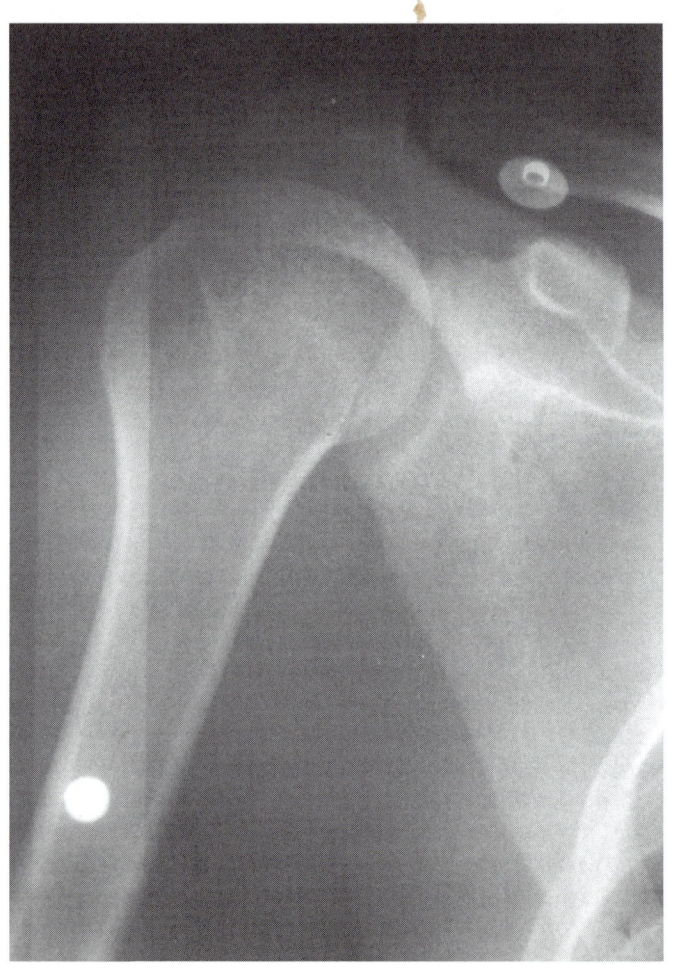

Case F

B. S., a 30-year-old grave digger, was preparing a burial vault. As he lifted the heavy granite cover, he lost his balance, and the heavy cover fell back on his right hand. He was unable to return to work because of pain and swelling in the hand.

1. *The x-ray (Figure F-1) shows*
    a) no abnormality of the carpal bones.
    b) a nondisplaced fracture of the triquetrum.
    c) an old fracture of the hamate.
    d) grade II–III scapholunate dissociation.
    e) a fracture of the carpal scaphoid (navicular).

2. *This patient*
    a) should be admitted for urgent operative repair.
    b) should be placed in a cast or splint that incorporates the thumb.
    c) should be told that healing of this fracture will be no problem.
    d) should be given an ACE bandage and returned for follow-up in 2 to 5 days.
    e) should be returned to work and told he does not need narcotics for pain.

3. *Possible complications from this accident include*
    a) forearm compartment syndrome.
    b) median nerve compression (carpal tunnel).
    c) osteonecrosis of the fractured bone.
    d) nonunion (delayed union).
    e) all of the above, which can cause pain and disability.

Answers: 1. e), 2. b), 3. e).

FIGURE F-1 Injury film in Case F.

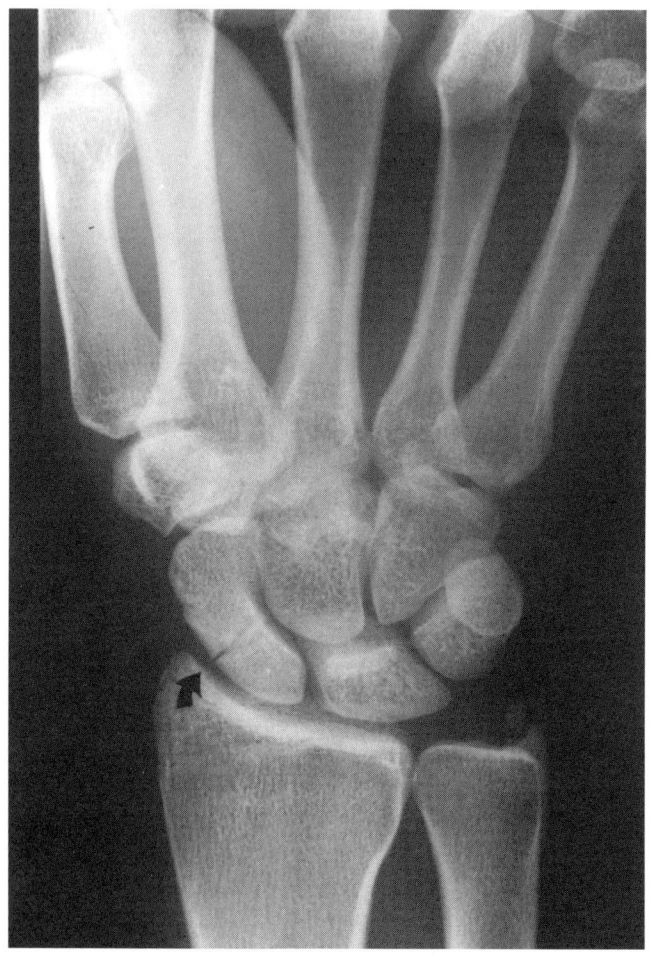

Discussion:

Scaphoid fractures are problem fractures. The reasons are that the mechanical forces to displacement are high and the blood supply to the proximal pole of the scaphoid is retrograde. Even apparently nondisplaced fractures can have a complicated course. It is helpful to explain these facts from the outset, because many of the patients sustaining this injury work with their hands and can lose their livelihood and way in the world. Long periods of casting, operative repair, bone grafting, and electrical stimulation of bone healing are some of the treatment options. Since a heavy stone fell on the patient's hand he may experience additional complications from the crush injury.

Case G

A 43-year-old woman was headed downstairs. She turned at the landing and fell, hurting her ankle. In the emergency department x-rays were taken of her deformed and swollen ankle (Figures G-1, G-2).

1. *This is an injury that should be*
   a) splinted as is and referred in 2 to 3 days to an orthopedist.
   b) splinted as is and referred within 2 to 3 hours to an orthopedist.
   c) reduced, splinted, and released with crutches and pain medication.
   d) reduced, splinted, and hospitalized for probable treatment under anesthesia.
   e) sent for immediate angiography to rule out arterial injury.

2. *In this trimalleolar fracture the following structures are broken:*
   a) the medial (here the deltoid ligament) and lateral malleoli.
   b) the anteroinferior tib-fib ligament.
   c) the posterior malleolus.
   d) (a) and (c).
   e) (a), (b), & (c).

3. *The x-ray shows*
   a) a spiral fracture of the fibula.
   b) a double fracture of the fibula.
   c) a comminuted fracture of the fibula.
   d) an adduction fracture of the medial malleolus.
   e) a fracture of the tibial plafond.

FIGURE G-1 Lateral x-ray of the injured ankle in Case G.

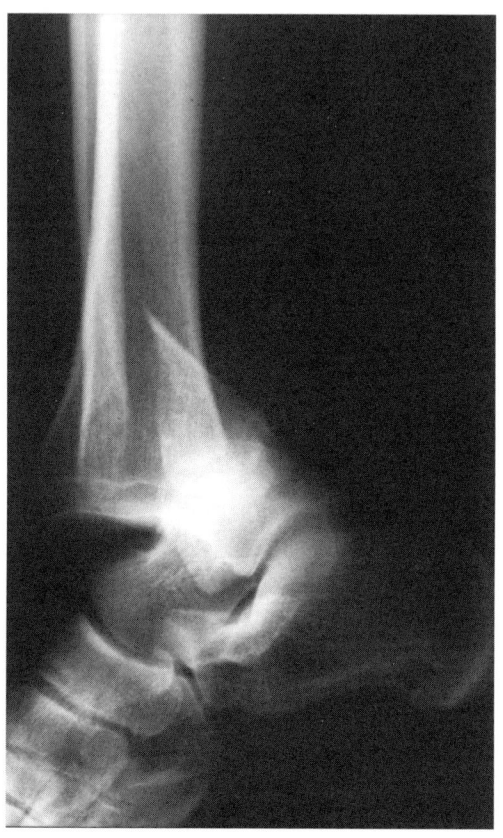

CASE G 209

FIGURE G-2 AP x-ray in Case G.

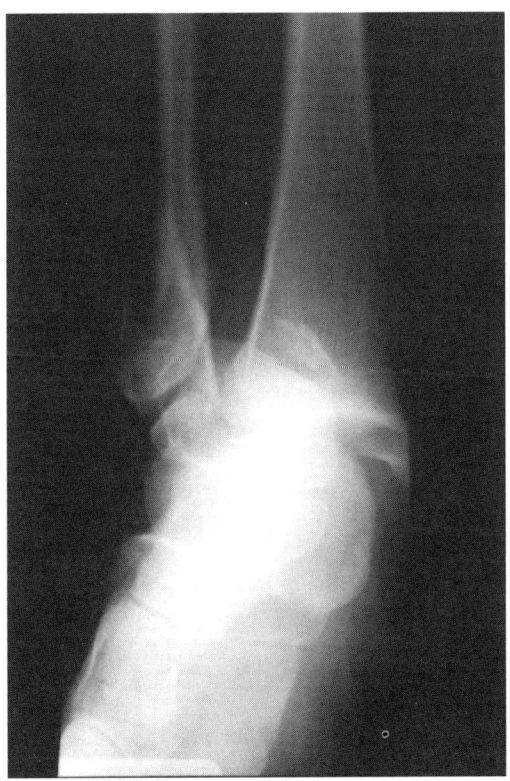

4. *Reduction and splinting in the ER*
   a) should not be attempted.
   b) wastes time—the patient needs urgent surgery.
   c) is risky; the fracture may compound.
   d) reduces pain, protects the skin.
   e) may damage the skin and cause swelling and blisters.

Answers: 1. d), 2. e), 3. a), 4. d).

Discussion:

Trimalleolar-fracture dislocations can be treated by closed reduction and casting or by operative repair with stabilization of the fibula and the medial malleolus. In either treatment, the talus should be replaced beneath the tibia with the fibula at full length (Figures G-3, G-4). Hospitalization is required. The ankle may become swollen, and fracture blisters are common. The results of treatment are usually good. However, both operative and nonoperative treatments can be complicated by thromboembolism, skin problems, and ankle arthrosis.

CASE G 211

FIGURE G-3 Postoperative lateral x-ray with fibula plate.

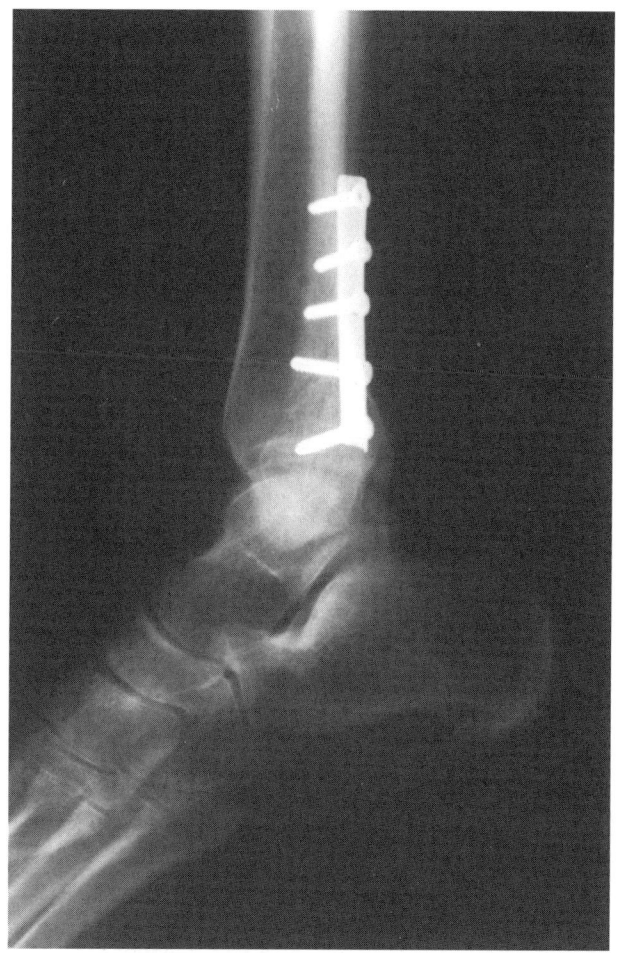

FIGURE G-4 Postoperative AP x-ray shows the talus centered in the mortise.

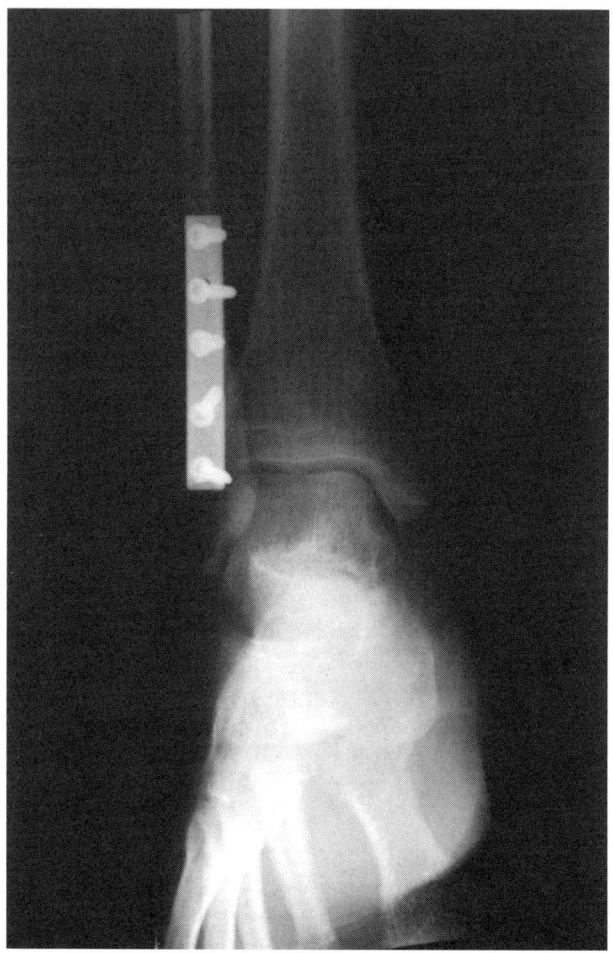

Case H

O. H., an 86-year-old man, fell from a chair in the nursing home while leaning over to a neighbor. He had adult-onset diet-controlled diabetes, mild hypertension for which he was taking a diuretic, slight cardiac irregularity, and prostatism. Physical examination revealed a shortened, externally rotated left thigh, which was painful to manipulate, and a bruise over the greater trochanter.

1. *The most likely diagnosis is*
   a) dislocated left hip.
   b) pelvic ring fracture (Malgaigne type).
   c) intertrochanteric fracture of the left hip.
   d) a left femoral neck fracture.
   e) a left femoral shaft fracture.

2. *The most likely diagnosis is confirmed by x-ray. (See Figure H-1). Definitive treatment of this fracture will be accomplished by*
   a) some form of internal fixation.
   b) external skeletal fixation.
   c) skeletal or skin traction.
   d) a 1½ spika plaster cast.
   e) bedrest and early functional mobilization.

3. *Initial assessment should include*
   a) CBC, chemistries, and urinalysis.
   b) chest x-ray and EKG.
   c) Protime and PTT; type and crossmatch.
   d) all of the above
   e) selected laboratory examination based on clinical findings.

FIGURE H-1 Injury x-ray in Case H.

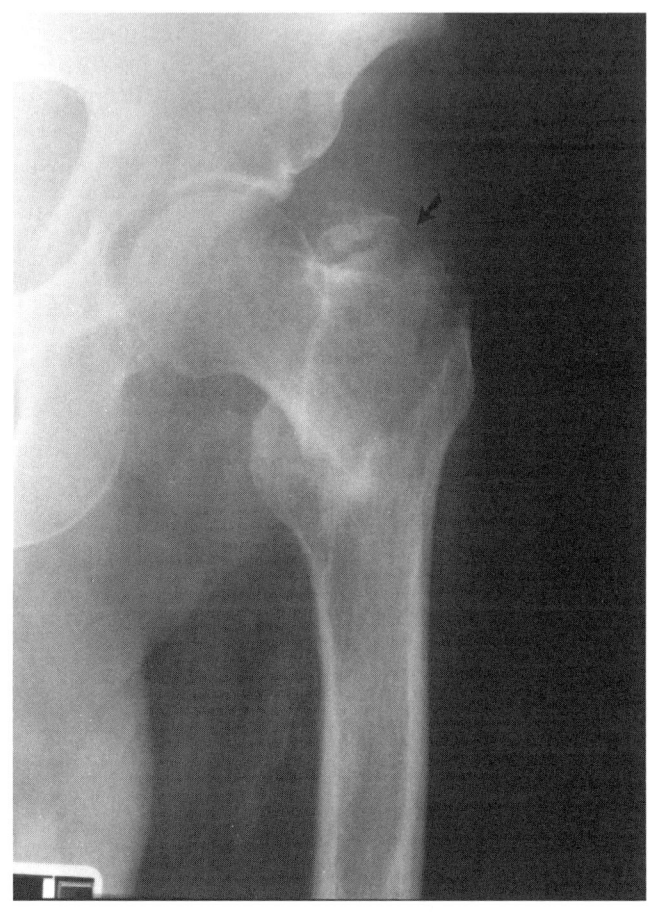

For questions 4 through 8 determine whether the statement is True or False.

4. This is a common injury in elderly patients. ____
5. This injury has an appreciable mortality. ____
6. Definitive treatment is not urgent. ____
7. Preoperative ambulatory status correlates with outcome. ____
8. The incidence of this fracture is rising. ____

Answers: 1. c), 2. a), 3. d), 4. T, 5. T, 6. F, 7. T, 8. T.

Discussion:

Elderly patients require early definitive operative treatment for hip fractures to prevent morbidity and preserve function. Falls are common in the elderly and, when associated with a hip fracture, are a common cause of hospitalization. Patients who were ambulatory before falling do better than those who were not. The incidence of this injury is rising. Urgent treatment with early postoperative ambulation lowers the rate of complications including pneumonia, bedsores, confusion, and thromboembolism (Figure H-2).

FIGURE H-2 Treatment with a sliding hip screw.

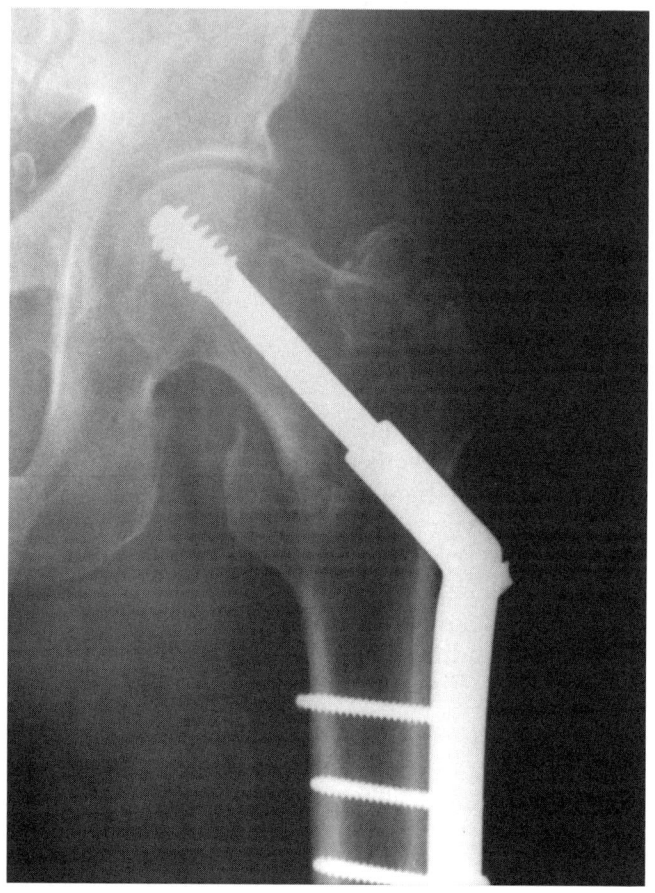

Case I

D. G., a 34-year-old welder, was driving his motorcycle when he hit a slick spot in a turn and was thrown at high speed into a tree, sustaining multiple injuries. At the scene he was hypotensive with a blood pressure of 70 and labored respirations. He was unresponsive to painful stimuli, but his pupils reacted to light. He was brought to the trauma station in the emergency department.

Place the immediate steps in his care in order of their priority.

a) Abdominal ultrasound.   1. ____
b) Cervical spine, chest, pelvis (single shot x-rays).   2. ____
c) Large-bore IV's, treatment of shock.   3. ____
d) Splinting of skeletal fractures.   4. ____
e) Intubation—airway management.   5. ____

6. *Injuries included a pelvis fracture, femur fracture, and humerus fracture. The abdominal ultrasound was negative. He was taken to x-ray for a CT of his head, which showed a skull fracture and cerebral contusion. The blood pressure could not be maintained despite four units of packed cells and four liters of Ringer's solution.*

    a) The head injury is responsible for his shock.
    b) Bleeding from the pelvis fracture may be the problem.
    c) He has a thoracic injury and is bleeding into his chest.
    d) Any of (a), (b), or (c) is possible.
    e) Blood incompatibility is the most likely cause of his failure to respond to therapy.

7. *The fracture of the pelvis (Figure I-1)*
    a) is a stable "open-book" type.
    b) is an unstable vertical shear fracture.

FIGURE I-1 Injury pelvis film in Case I.

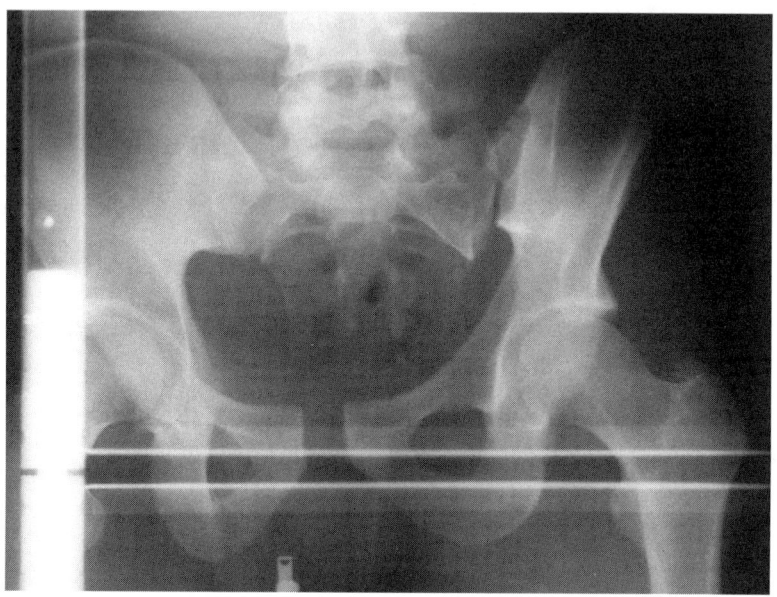

c) is a complex acetabular fracture-dislocation.
d) is a lateral compression fracture.
e) is a Malgaigne fracture.

For questions 8 through 12 determine whether the statement is True or False.

8. External skeletal fixation may help control bleeding. ____
9. Anteriography with embolization may help control bleeding. ____
10. Celiostomy with arterial ligation is the best way to control bleeding. ____
11. Bleeding from the pelvic fracture is unlikely to be prolonged. ____
12. External pelvic compression with a sling will help control bleeding. ____

Answers: 1. e), 2. c), 3. b), 4. a), 5. d), 6. d), 7. b), 8. T, 9. T, 10. F, 11. F, 12. F.

Discussion:

Polytrauma patients present with a constellation of complex problems. Priorities in care have been established and a surprising number of severely injured people saved. Severe cranial trauma and uncontrolled pelvic hemorrhage are two of the great challenges remaining in traumatology. A combination of limited skeletal stabilization with angiographic embolization of bleeding vessels appears to offer the best chance for survival. Unfortunately, in most hospitals angiography and the operating room are in different directions. Improved organization of trauma systems could save more lives.

Case J

D. Z., a 37-year-old woman, was stopped at a stop sign when she was rear-ended by a truck. Her car sustained minor damage. She initially felt all right and did not seek medical care. A week later she began to have neck stiffness, headaches, right shoulder pain, and tingling in her forearm and fingers. She sought care at the local emergency department. The past history revealed prior treatment for cervical malalignment with manipulation.

1. *Initial assessment should include*
    a) history and physical.
    b) plain cervical films and right shoulder x-ray.
    c) cervical CT.
    d) (a) and (b).
    e) (a), (b), and (c).

2. *The lateral cervical spine x-ray (Figure J-1) shows*
    a) a hangman's fracture.
    b) subluxation of C_2 on C_3.
    c) cervical disc space narrowing and degenerative changes at several levels.
    d) an acute cervical disc rupture.
    e) a large retropharyngeal hematoma.

3. *D. Z. should be told*
    a) the accident caused no damage.
    b) there are no new gross abnormalities that require hospitalization.
    c) to stop worrying and complaining about her neck.
    d) she has a neck fracture and will need hospitalization.
    e) to seek legal help.

FIGURE J-1 Lateral c-spine x-ray in Case J.

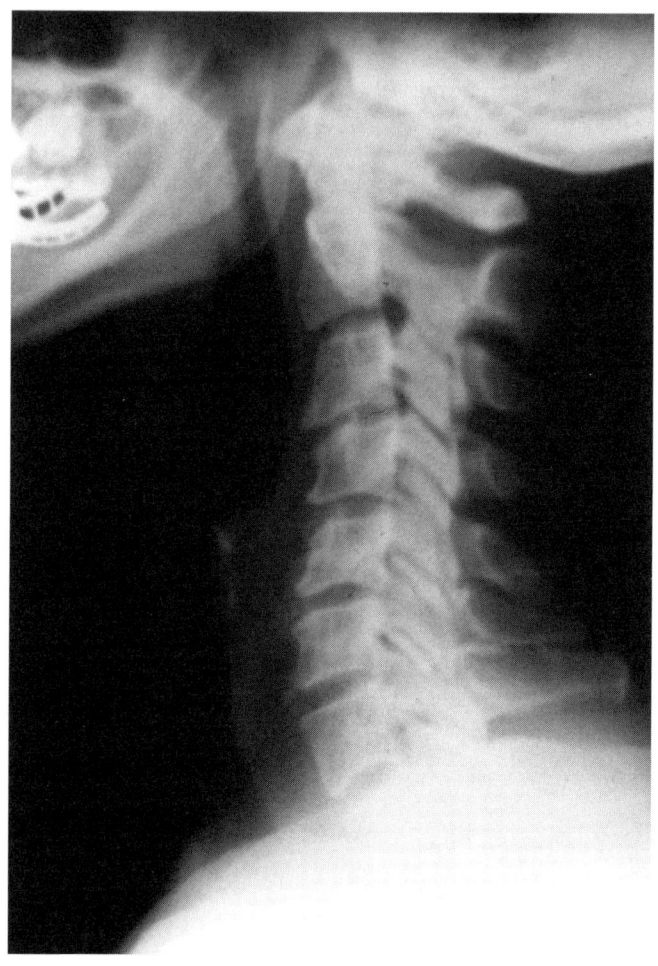

4. *Thoughtful disposition includes*
- **a)** pain medication.
- **b)** soft cervical collar.
- **c)** follow-up appointment.
- **d)** all of the above.
- **e)** none of the above.

Answers: 1. d), 2. c), 3. b), 4. d).

Discussion:

Injury to cervical motion segments—discs, facet joints, and surrounding ligaments and muscle—produce a cascade of symptoms with little objective evidence of damage. These patients feel hurt, and their anxiety—particularly when they are not properly examined and treated—amplifies the problem. It is sensible to document the history carefully. Consider that minor soft tissue injury can produce marked disability and arrange for a treatment program that will promote healing and prompt resolution of the effects of trauma.

CASE K

A. S., a 30-year-old man, was emerging from a bar when he leaped out of the way of an oncoming car and fell on his left arm. On evaluation in the emergency room, he had a painful deformed left elbow. An x-ray was taken (Figure K-1).

1. *The initial x-ray shows a posterior elbow dislocation. Physical examination should rule out:*
   a) disruption of the collateral ligaments.
   b) median, radial, or ulnar nerve palsy.
   c) Volkmann's contracture.
   d) all three of (a), (b), and (c).
   e) both (a) and (c).

2. *After reduction in the emergency room another x-ray was taken (Figure K-2). This x-ray shows:*
   a) the elbow is reduced; the patient can go home.
   b) the elbow is reduced; the patient needs a splint.
   c) the elbow is still dislocated; try another reduction.
   d) the elbow is still dislocated; try another reduction, this time under anesthesia.
   e) the elbow is subluxed; it will need an operative repair of torn collateral ligaments.

Match the acute complicating nerve palsy with the dislocated joint:

3. Shoulder   a. Ulna
4. Elbow   b. Sciatic
5. Hip   c. Axillary
6. Knee   d. Peroneal

FIGURE K-1 Initial x-ray showing a posterior elbow dislocation.

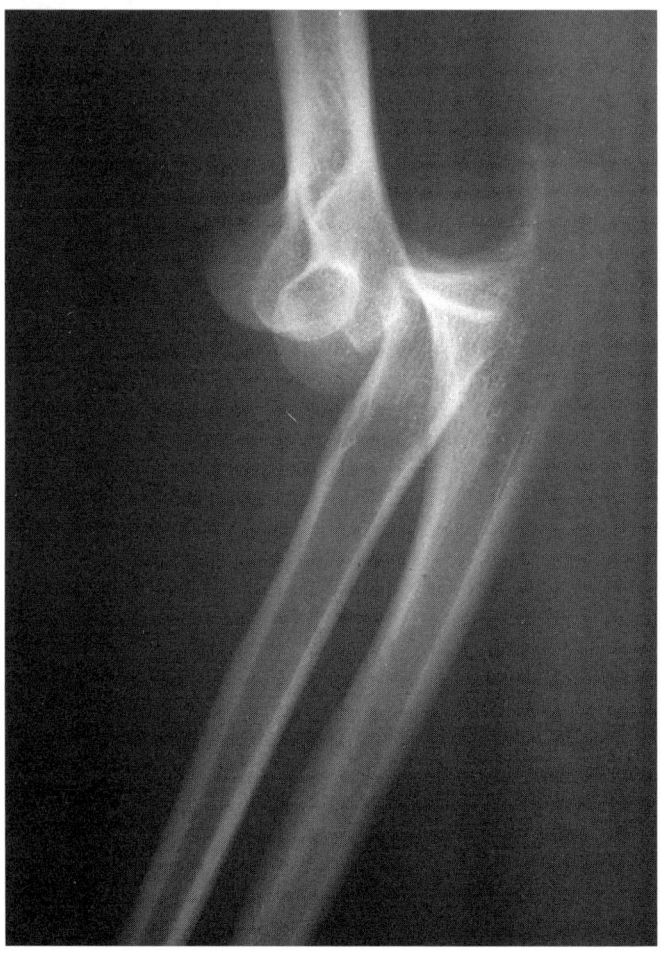

FIGURE K-2 X-ray taken after reduction.

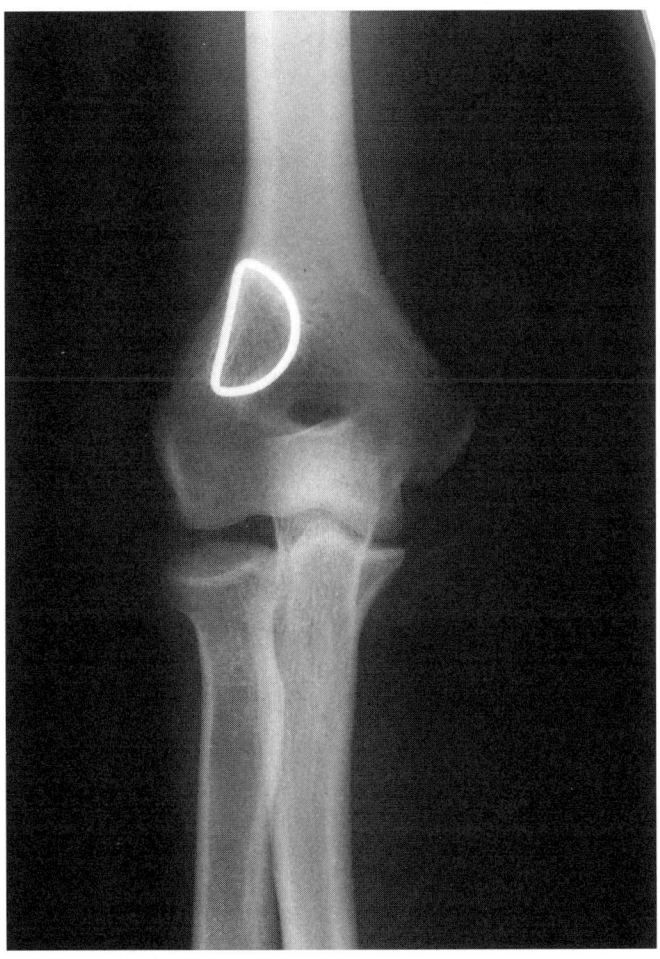

Match the chronic complication with the dislocated joint:

7. Shoulder	a.	Loss of range of motion
8. Elbow	b.	Osteonecrosis
9. Hip	c.	Ligamentous laxity
10. Knee	d.	Recurrent dislocation

Answers: 1. d), 2. e), 3. c), 4. a), 5. b), 6. d), 7. d), 8. a), 9. b), 10. c).

Discussion:

Dislocated joints are always accompanied by torn ligaments. The origins and/or insertions of ligaments can be torn off, and then so-called "avulsion fractures" are seen on x-ray. Alternatively, the ligaments are torn in midsubstance, and no bone fragments are visible on x-ray. Ligamentous healing is not perfect, so, depending on the joint involved, completely normal function is seldom the end result. Furthermore, as the joint separates, its surfaces may bump, causing cartilage fragments to break off. Those fragments, along with the residual discrepancies in joint tracking, set the stage for late joint degeneration—arthrosis. This complication is more likely than not after dislocation of a major joint.

SUGGESTED READINGS

Bone Physiology

Bourne GH, (ed). The biochemistry and physiology of bone. New York: Academic Press, 1972.

Brighton CT. Principles of fracture healing (part I). American Academy of Orthopedic Surgery. Instructional Course Lectures. Vol. XXXIII, pp. 60–82, 1984.

Brighton CT. Principles of fracture healing (part II). American Academy of Orthopedic Surgery. Instructional Course Lectures. Vol. XXXIII, pp. 82–106, 1984.

Brighton CT, Buckwalter JA, Cooper RR, et al. Physiology of bone. American Academy of Orthopedic Surgery. Instructional Course Lectures. Vol. XXXVI, pp. 1–86, 1987.

Inflammatory Processes

Dvorkin ML. Office orthopedics. Norwalk CT: Appleton & Lange, 1993.

McCarty, Koopman WJ, eds. Arthritis and allied conditions. Philadelphia: Lea & Febiger, 1993.

Huskisson EC, Hart FD: Joint disease: all the arthropathies. Bristol Wright, 1987.

Musculoskeletal Radiology

Harris JH, Harris WH, Novelline, eds. The radiology of emergency medicine. Baltimore: Williams & Wilkins, 1993.

Rosen P, Doris PE, Barkin RM, et al., eds. Diagnostic radiology in emergency medicine. St. Louis: Mosby Yearbook, 1992.

Polytrauma

Gill W, Long III WB: Shock trauma manual. Baltimore: Williams & Wilkins, 1979.

Meyers MH, ed. The multiply injured patient with complex fractures. Philadelphia: Lea & Febiger, 1984.

Richardson JD, Polk HC, Flint LM, eds. Trauma: clinical care and pathophysiology. Chicago: Year Book Medical Publishers, 1987.

Zuidema GD, Rutherford RB, Bullinger WF, eds. The management of trauma. Philadelphia: W.B. Saunders, 1985.

Fractures

Browner BD, Jupiter JB, Levine AM, Trofton PG, eds. Skeletal trauma. Philadelphia: W.B. Saunders, 1992.

Crenshaw AH, ed. Campbell's operative orthopaedics. St. Louis: Mosby, 1992.

Rockwood CA, Green DP, eds. Fractures in adults. New York: J.B. Lippincott, Vols. 1 and 2, 1993.

Schatzker J, Tile M. The rationale of operative fracture care. Berlin: Springer-Verlag, 1987.

Pediatric Fractures

Green NE, Swiontkowski MF, eds. Skeletal trauma in children. Philadelphia: W.B. Saunders, 1992.

Griffin PP, Hamilton CM. Fractures in children. American Academy of Orthopedic Surgery. Instructional Course Lectures. Vol. XIX, pp. 150–171, 1970.

Ogden JA. Pocket guide to pediatric fractures. Baltimore: Williams & Wilkins, 1987.

Rockwood CA, Green DP, King RE, eds. Fractures in children. New York: J.B. Lippincott, Vol. 3, 1993.

Staheli LT. Fundamentals of pediatric orthopedics. New York: Raven Press, 1992.

Casts and Traction

Chadnofsky CR, Otten EJ, Newmeyer WL. Splinting techniques. In: Roberts JR, Hedges JR, eds. Clinical procedures in emergency medicine: Philadelphia: W.B. Saunders, pp. 782–809, 1991.

Freuler F, Weidmer U, Bianchini D. Cast manual for adults and children. Berlin: Springer-Verlag, 1979.

Lewis RC, Jr. Handbook of traction, casting and splinting techniques. Philadelphia: J.B. Lippincott, 1977.

Salib PI. Plaster casting. New York: Appleton-Century-Crofts, 1975.

External and Internal Fixation

Browner BD, Edwards CC, eds. The science and practice of intramedullary nailing. Philadelphia: Lea & Febiger, 1987.

Coombs R, Green S, Sarmiento A, eds. External fixation and functional bracing. London: Orthotext, 1989.

Seligson D, ed. Concepts in intramedullary nailing. New York: Grune & Stratton, 1985.

Seligson D, Pope M, eds. Concepts in external fixation. New York: Grune & Stratton, 1982.

Spine

Cailliet R. Low back pain syndrome. Philadelphia: FA Davis Co., 1988.

Errico TJ, Bauer RD, Waugh T, eds. Spinal trauma. Philadelphia: J.B. Lippincott, 1991.

Galli RL, Spaite DW, Simon RR, eds. Emergency orthopedics: the spine. Norwalk, CT: Appleton & Lange, 1989.

Herkowitz HN, Garfin SR, Balderston RA, et al., eds. The spine. Philadelphia: W. B. Saunders, 1992.

Shoulder

Lippert FG. Shoulder pain. In: Decision making in emergency medicine, Callahan, Barton, and Schumaker, eds. Philadelphia: B.C. Decker, Inc., pp. 290–291, 1990.

Rowe CR, ed. The shoulder. New York: Churchill Livingston, 1988.

Elbow

Tullos HS, Schwab G, Bennett JB, et al. Fractures about the elbow. American Academy of Orthopedic Surgery. Instructional Course Lectures. Vol. XXX, pp. 185–238, 1981.

Wrist

Gelberman RH, ed. The wrist. New York: Raven Press, 1994.

Gilula LA, ed. The traumatized hand and wrist. Philadelphia: W.B. Saunders, 1992.

Lichtman DM, ed. The wrist and its disorders. Philadelphia: W.B. Saunders, 1988.

Taleisnik J. Wrist: anatomy, function, and injury. American Academy of Orthopedic Surgery. Instructional Course Lectures. Vol. XXVII, pp. 61–87, 1978.

Hand

Ariyan S. The hand book. New York: McGraw Hill, 1989.

Jupiter JB, ed. Flynn's hand surgery. Baltimore: Williams & Wilkins, 1991.

Lamb DW, Hooper G, Kuczynski K, eds. The practice of hand surgery. Oxford: Blackwell Scientific Publications.

Milford L. The hand. St. Louis: Mosby, 1988.

Troublesome fractures and dislocations of the hand. American Academy of Orthopedic Surgery. Instructional Course Lectures. Vol. XIX, pp. 130–149, 1970.

Pelvic and Acetabular Fractures

Emerson RH, Lhowe DW. Fractures of the pelvis. In: May HL, ed. Emergency medicine. Boston: Little, Brown, & Co., 1992.

Kane JW. Fractures of the pelvis. American Academy of Orthopedic Surgery. Instructional Course Lectures. Vol. XXVIII, pp. 1–6, 1979.

Schatzker J, Tile M. The rationale of operative fracture care. Berlin: Springer-Verlag, 1987.

Hip

Massie WK. Fractures of the hip. American Academy of Orthopedic Surgery. Instructional Course Lectures. Vol. XVIII, J2, 1962–69.

Meyers MH, ed. Fractures of the hip. Chicago: Year Book Medical Publishers, 1985.

Tronzo RG, ed. Surgery of the hip joint. New York: Springer-Verlag, 1984.

Knee

Fu FH, ed. Knee surgery. Baltimore: Williams & Wilkins, 1994.

Insall JN, ed. Surgery of the knee. Baltimore: Williams & Wilkins, 1994.

Larson RL, Grana WA, eds. The knee: form, function, pathology, and treatment. Philadelphia: W.B. Saunders, 1993.

Scott WN, ed. The knee. St. Louis: Mosby, 1994.

Ankle

Hamilton WC, ed. Traumatic disorders of the ankle. New York: Springer-Verlag, 1984.

Johnson KA, ed. The foot and ankle. New York: Raven Press, 1984.

Rosen P, Barkin RM, eds. Emergency medicine concepts and clinical practice. St. Louis: Mosby Yearbook, pp. 745–777, 1992.

Foot

Gould JS, Thompson FM, Cracchiolo III A, et al., eds. Operative foot surgery. Philadelphia: W.B. Saunders, 1994.

Helal B, Wilson D, eds. The foot. London: Churchill Livingston, 1988.

Mann RA, Coughlin MJ, eds. Surgery of the foot and ankle. St. Louis: Mosby, 1993.

McGlamry ED, Banks AS, Downey MS, eds. Comprehensive textbook of foot surgery. Baltimore: Williams & Wilkins, 1992.

INDEX

Page numbers followed by (*t*) indicate tables, page numbers followed by (*f*) indicate figures.

Abbreviated injury scale (AIS), 14-15, 15*t*
Acetabular fractures, 103-107
 See also Pelvic fractures
Achilles' tendon, 34
ACL. *See* Anterior cruciate ligament
Acromioclavicular separation, 63, 65*f*, 68*t*
 severe (grade III), 64*f*
Acromion, 63
Acute low back pain, 174-177
 lumbar spine conditions, 176*t*
 pinched nerve
  nerve conduction, 175-176
  nerve root irritation, 175-176
 sciatic scoliosis, 175
 spondylolithesis, 176
AIS. *See* Abbreviated injury scale
Amputations, compound fractures, 18, 21*f*
Anesthesia
 in pain management, 44-45
Ankle dislocation, 157
Ankle fractures, 146
 ankle mortise, 146
 high-grade fracture, 149, 150*f*
 Lauge-Hansen classification, 147
 radiographic evaluation, 147, 148*f*
 Weber classification of fibula fractures, 147, 149*t*

Ankle injuries, 145-153
 fractures, 146-150
 pilon fractures, 151-153
 sprains, 145-146
Ankle sprains
 evaluating anterotalofibular ligament, 145-146
 ligamentous injury types, 145
Anterior cruciate ligament (ACL), 123
Anterior dislocation of shoulder, 67, 68*t*
Anterior drawer test, 134
Anterior spinal artery syndrome, 165
Arms neurologic function testing of, 14
Arthritis, 33
Arthrosis 33, 66
Assess, cleanse, treat (ACT) of open-compound fractures, 19
Avascular necrosis, 3
Avulsion fracture, 100
Axial traction, 67
 dislocated elbow and, 77

Barton's fracture, 3
Baseball fracture, 97
Bending fracture of humerus shaft, 72*f*
Bennett's fracture, 97

235

INDEX

Biceps tendinitis, 68
Biceps tendon, 34
Bipartite patella, 129, 130f
Bone
  callus, 27, 30
  fracture and hematoma, 27
  healing
    primary, 30
    secondary, 30
  healing time, 27, 28f
    long, 27
  inspection
    fracture pattern, 10, 11f
    location of fracture, 9-10
Bone remodeling, 27, 30
Boutonniere deformity, 100
Boxer's fracture, 3, 97, 98-99f
Brachial plexus, 63
Buckle fracture, 6
Buck's traction, 53, 54
Bursa, 34
Bursitis, 33, 35
Burst fracture, 3

Calcaneal apophysitis, 34t
Calcaneus and talus fractures and dislocations, 157-158
Calcific tendinitis, 35
Calcium salts, 34
Callus, 27, 30
Capital femoral epiphysitis, 34t
Capitate, 91f, 93
Capitellum, radial head, internal epicondyle, trochlea, olecranon, external epicondyle (CRiTOe), 77, 78
Carpel tunnel syndrome, 88t
Carpo-metacarpal arthritis of thumb, 88t
Casts, 37-39, 41
  fiberglass casting, 41t
  "hanging arm cast," 71
  plaster-of-Paris casting, 41t
Causalgias, 44
Cephalosporin, 48

Cervical radiculopathy, 68
Cervical spine fractures and dislocations, 166-171
  cervical spine immobilization, 168t
  immobilize, radiograph, assess, 166
  lateral cervical spine x-ray, 171, 172f
  quick assessment of motor function of conscious patient, 168t
  suspect neck injury, 166, 167f
  unstable spine, 169, 170f
Cervical spine immobilization, 168t
Chance (slice) fracture, 3
Circular solid casts, 39
Circulation, lack of, 25
Clavicle, 63
Clavicle fractures, 40f, 63, 64f, 65f, 66, 68t
Closed fracture, 3
Coaptation splint, 71
Colles' fracture, 3
  distal radius fractures, 90
Comminuted fracture, 3, 10, 11f
Compartment syndrome, 25, 84
Complex comminuted fracture, 10, 11f
  of tibia, 29f
Compound fracture, 3, 17-18, 19f
  of tibia, 29f
Compression fracture, 4
Contamination
  open injury and, 18
Coracoid, 63
Corticosteroids, 34
Costochondral junction, inflammation of, 34t
Costochondritis, 34t
CRiTOe mnemonic. See Capitellum, radial head, internal epicondyle, trochlea, olecranon, external epicondyle
Cruciate ligament, 123

Débridement
  open fracture and, 17, 20f
Definitive treatment of simple fractures, 37, 39, 40t
Delayed union, 71
DeQuervain's disease, 8, 88t
Diaphyseal cortex-to-cortex fractures, 158
Diaphyseal fractures, 11f
DIP. *See* Distal interphalangeal
Dislocation, 4
  elbow, acute, 24f
  hip, 117-118
  intercarpal, 93
  knee, 131-137
  of major joint, 23, 24f
  shoulder, 63, 67-68, 68t
  of humeral head, 65f
Displaced fractures, operative repair of, 47
Distal femur and proximal tibia fractures, 124-128
  children's patterns of injury, 125
  Osgood-Schlatter's disease, 125
  pediatric epiphyseal injuries, 128f
  Pellegrini-Steada disease, 125
  Segond fractures, 124
  supracondylar fractures, 124
  tibial plateau fractures, 125, 126-127f
Distal interphalangeal (DIP), 96
Distal radioulnar joint (DRUJ), 85
Distal radius, nonarticular fracture of, 92f
DRUJ. *See* Distal radioulnar joint

Ecchymosis, 48
Elbow, acute dislocation of, 24f
Elbow injuries, 77
  axial traction, 77
  capitellum, 77
  CRiTOe mnemonic for order of epiphyses appearance, 77, 78
  displaced fracture, 78, 79f
  external epicondyle, 77
  internal epicondyle, 77
  Little League elbow, 77
  Monteggia's fracture, 78
  olecranon, 77
  radial head, 77
  stockbroker's elbow, 77
  tennis elbow, 77
  trochlea, 77
  Volkmann's ischemic contracture, 78
  x-ray, 80f
Embolism syndrome, 122
Epiphyseal-diaphyseal fracture, 128f
Epiphyseal slip, 128f
  with metaphyseal fragment, 128f
Epiphyses appearance, order of, CRiTOe mnemonic, 77, 78
Epiphysitis of capitellum, 34t
Examination, importance of, 7-8
ExFix (external fixateur). *See* External fixateur
Extensor tendon, 34
External fixateur, 4, 14, 50, 51f
  half pins, 50
  on humerus, 73f
  pain and, 52
  problems caused by pin tracts, 50
  thin wires (Kirschner or K-wires), 50
  of tibia, 20f, 29f
  transfixing pins, 50
External rotation(s)
  of abducted arm, 67
  order of insertion, 67
Extracapsular fractures, 110, 115

Fasciitis, 33
Fat embolism syndrome, 122
  treatment of, 122
Floating knee, 120
Femoral shaft fractures, 119

Femoral shaft fractures, (continued)
  common problems after femur fracture, 122
  embolism syndrome, 122
  emergent treatment, 120
  fat embolism syndrome, 122
    treatment of, 122
  floating knee, 120
  fracture pattern, complexity, location, 120, 121f
  long spiral fractures, 120
  transverse fractures, 120
Fiberglass casting, 41t
Fibrocartilage, 33
Figure-of-eight soft clavicle straps, 66
Flexor carpi ulnaris, 35
Foot fractures, 155
  ankle dislocation, 157
  common fractures, 156t
  diaphyseal cortex-to-cortex fractures, 158
  fractures and dislocations
    forefoot, 158-161
    talus and calcaneus, 157-158
  hallux valgus, 158
  Jones' fracture, 158, 159-160f
  metatarsal phalangeal joint (MTP), 161
  metatarsus adductus, 158
  pantalar dislocation, 157
  subtalar dislocation, 157
Forearm fractures, 83-85
  compartment syndrome, 84
  distal radioulnar joint (DRUJ), 85
  evaluating neurologic function, 83
  Galeazzi's, 83
  greenstick, 84
  Monteggia's, 83
  night-stick, 83
  parry, 83
  plate fixation treatment, 84
  Volkmann's contracture, 84

Forefoot fractures and dislocations, 158-161
Fracture(s)
  acetabulum, 103-107
  ankle, 146-150
  avulsion, 100
  Barton's, 3
  boxer's, 3
  buckle, 6
  burst, 3
  chance (slice), 3
  closed, 3
  Colles', 3
  comminuted, 3, 10, 11f
  complex, 10, 11f
  compound, 3
  compression, 4
  distal femur and proximal tibia, 124-129
  elbow, 77
  epiphyseal-diaphyseal, 128f
  femoral shaft, 119
  foot, 155-161
  forearm, 83-85
  Galeazzi's, 4, 83
  green stick, 4, 6, 84
  hand, 95-97
  hangman's, 4
  hip, 109-117
  Hoffa's, 124
  of humerus shaft, 69-75
  intercarpal, 93
  Jefferson's, 4
  Jones', 4
  leg, 139-144
  Lisfranc's fracture-dislocation, 4
  Malgaigne's, 4
  Monteggia's, 4, 83
  night-stick, 5, 83
  oblique, 10, 11f
  open, 5
  parry, 5, 83
  patella, 129-131
  pathologic, 5
  pelvic, 103-107
  pilon, 5, 151-153

Segond's, 5
of shoulder, 63, 64f, 65f, 68t
  clavicle, 66, 68t
  proximal humerus, 66
  scapula, 66
simple, 5, 10, 11f
Smith's, 5
spine, 163-171
spiral, 10, 11f, 69
straddle, 6
thoracolumbar, 171-174
torus, 6
trans-epiphyseal, 128f
transverse, 10, 11f
wrist, 87-93
Fracture emergencies, 23, 24f, 25
  lack of circulation, 25
  progressive loss of neurologic function, 23
  progressive pain, paralysis, pallor, pulselessness in limb (compartment syndrome), 25
  unreduced dislocation of major joint, 23, 24f
Fracture treatment, 30
Frankel's grades below a transverse lesion, 165t

Galeazzi's fracture, 4, 83
Gardner-Wells tongs, 54
Gluteus medius tendon, 35
Grade I, II, III sprain, 8t
Greater tuberosity fracture, 65f, 66
Green stick fracture, 4, 6, 84

Half pins, 50
Hamate, 93
Hand fractures, 95
  baseball fracture, 97
  Bennett's fracture, 97
  boxer's fracture, 97, 98-99f
  distal interphalangeal (DIP), 96
  mallet finger, 97
  proximal interphalangeal (PIP), 96
  swan-neck deformity, 97
"Hanging arm cast," 71
Hangman's fracture, 4
Healing times, 28f
  adult skin, 27
  bone remodeling, 27
  ligaments, 27
  long bones, 27
  muscle-tendon units, 27
  scar maturation, 27
  tendons, 27
Hematoma
  bone fracture and, 27
Hemisection of cord, 165
Hemorrhage
  pelvic fractures and, 103, 105, 106-107f
Hip dislocations, 117-118
Hip fractures, 109-115, 116f
  accident-painful hip, 111f
  displaced fracture, 110, 114f
  extracapsular fractures, 110, 115
  intertrochanteric fractures, 115
  intracapsular fractures, 110, 112-113f
  problems following hip-fracture fixation in elderly, 117t
  subtrochanteric fractures, 115
  x-rays, 110
History taking, 7-8
Hoffa fractures, 124
Humerus, 63
Humerus shaft, fractures of, 69
  bending fracture of, 72f
  coaptation splint, 71
  delayed union, 71
  examining for, recording radial nerve function, 69
  accident-painful arm, 70f
  external fixateur on, 73f
  geometry, 69
  "hanging arm cast," 71
  location, 69
  nonunion, 71

Humerus shaft, fractures of, (continued)
  pseudoarthrosis, 71
  radial nerve injury, 69
  sandwich splint, 71
  spiral fractures, 69
  well-healed fracture of, 74f
Hyaline cartilage, 33

Infection
  open fracture and, 17
Inflammation, 33
  of costochondral junction, 34t
  of joint, 33
  of pubic symphysis, 34t
Injury severity score (ISS), 15t
  equation for, 15
Intercarpal fractures and dislocations, 93
Internal derangement of knee, 135
Internal fixation. See Open reduction and internal fixation
Intertrochanteric fractures, 115
Intra-articular fractures, operative repair of, 47
Intracapsular fractures, 110, 112-113f
Intramedullary nailing, 14
Intramedullary nails, 47-48
  possible problems, 48
ISS. See Injury severity score

Jefferson's fracture, 4
Joint(s), examining, 10
  unreduced dislocation of major, 23
Jones' fracture, 4, 158, 159-160f

Kefzol (antibiotic), 17
Keinboch-Preisler disease, 88t
Kirschner or K-wires (thin wires), 50, 55
Knee injuries, 123-124
  accident-painful knee, 132-133f
  anterior cruciate ligament (ACL), 123
  anterior drawer test, 134
  dislocations, 131-137
    of tibia, 135, 136f
  internal derangement of knee, 135
  Lachmann test, 134
  ligamentous injuries, 131-137
  MacMurray's test, 135
  passive range of motion, 132, 133f
  posterior cruciate ligament (PCL), 123
  posterior drawer test, 134
  soft tissues of knee, 131t

LAC. See Long arm cast
Lachmann test, 134
Lauge-Hansen classification, 147
Legal and economic aspects of musculoskeletal injury, 57-59
  discovery phase of, 58
  malpractice, 59
  ramifications of, 58
Leg fractures, 139-144
  accident-painful leg, 140f
  displaced fractures, 139
  operative treatment, 141
    insertion of intramedullary nail, 142f
  overuse syndromes, 141, 143-144f
  patellar tendon bearing cast (PTB), 139
  stress fractures, 141, 143-144f
  tib-fib fracture, 139
Legg-Calvé-Perthes disease, 34t
Legs, neurologic function testing of, 14
Ligament(s)
  healing, 30
  healing time, 27
Ligament damage, 8t
Ligamentous injuries of knee, 131-137
  soft tissues of knee, 131t

INDEX   **241**

Lisfranc's fracture-dislocation, 4
Little Leaguer's elbow, 34t, 77
LLC. *See* Long leg cast
Long arm cast (LAC), 4
Long leg cast (LLC), 4
Long spiral fractures, 120
Lower limb traction, 55
Lunate, 93
'Lytic cocktail', 45

MacMurray's test, 135
Malgaigne's fracture, 4, 105
Mallet finger, 4, 97, 100
Malunion, 4
MAST trousers, 105
Medial meniscectomy of knee, 33
Meniscectomy, 4
Monteggia's fracture, 4, 78, 83
Morphine
  in pain management, 44
Muscle-tendon units
  healing time, 27, 28f
Musculoskeletal injury(ies)
  economic and legal aspects of, 57-59
    discovery phase, 58
    malpractice, 59
    ramifications of, 58
  immobilization, 37
  polytrauma and, 13-14
  three phases of emergent care of, 44
  treatment of, 27
Musculoskeletal pain, 43, 44t
Musculoskeletal shoulder problems, 68
Myoclonic jerks, 52

Narcotics
  advantages/disadvantages in pain management, 44-45
Nerve conduction, 175-176
Nerve root irritation, 175-176
Neurologic function, progressive loss of, 23

Night-stick fracture, 5, 83
Nonoperative (conservative bone treatment, 30
Nontransfixing traction, 54
Nonunion, 4, 71
Non-weight-bearing (NWB), 5
NWB. *See* Non-weight-bearing

Oblique fracture, 10, 11f
Open fracture, 5, 17-18, 19-21f
  antibiotic therapy for, 17
  assess, cleanse, treat (ACT), 19
  grade I, II, or III wound sizing, 17-18
  infection control of, 17
  priorities in treatment of, 17
  traumatic amputations, 18, 21f
Open reduction internal fixation (ORIF), 5, 48, 84
  clavicle fractures, 66
  of midshaft fractures, 49f
Operative repair for fracture treatment, 30, 47-48
  external fixateur, 51f
  open reduction and internal fixation of midshaft fractures, 49f
  strategies for, 47
ORIF. *See* Open reduction internal fixation
Orthopedic instrumentation, 47-52
Orthopedic problem solving components, 7
Orthopedic terminology, 3-6
Osgood-Schlatter's disease, 5, 34t, 125
Osteitis pubis, 34t
Osteochondroses, 33
  common, 34t
Osteophytes, 33
Osteosynthesis, 5, 14, 48
Overuse syndromes, 141, 143-144f

Pain, 43
  causalgias, 44

Pain, (continued)
  definition of, 43
  and external fixateurs, 52
  local anesthesia, 44-45
  'lytic cocktail', 45
  musculoskeletal, 43, 44t
  narcotic medications, use of, 44, 45
  and orthopedic injury, 52
  orthopedic measures, pain reducing, 44
  phantom limb, 44
  somatic, 43
  visceral, 43
Pain control for injury, 45t
Pain reducing orthopedic measures, 44
Pantalar dislocation, 157
Parry fracture, 5, 83
Partial-weight-bearing (PWB), 5
Patella fractures, 129-131
  bipartite patella, 129, 130f
  extensor mechanism of knee, 130f
  patella alta, 129
  patella baja, 129
Patellar tendon bearing cast (PTB), 139
Pathologic fracture, 5
PCL. *See* Posterior cruciate ligament
Pearson attachment, 55
PEEP. *See* Positive end expiratory pressure
Pelligrini-Steada disease, 125
Pelvic fractures, 103-107
  acetabular fractures, 103
  clinical signs of, 103
  control bleeding, 105, 106-107f
  Malgaigne's fracture, 105
  pelvic ring, 103
    hemorrhage, 103
  x-ray, 104f
Pelvic ring, 103
Penicillin
  open fracture antibiotic therapy, 17
Peritendinitis calcarea, 35, 88t
Phalen's test, 5
Phantom limb pain, 44
Pilon fracture, 5, 151-153
  distal tibial metaphysis, 151, 152f
  fibular fracture, 151
  grades of joint surface component, 151, 153
  "headset sign," 151
  open pilon fractures, 153
  syndesmosis rupture, 151
Pinched nerve, 175-176
PIP. *See* Proximal interphalangeal
Pisiform, 93
Plaster-of-Paris (POP), 5
Plaster-of-Paris casting, 41t
Plate-and-screw fixation, 47, 48
Polytrauma
  definition of, 13
  estimating severity of injury, 14-15
  high- and low-priority considerations in, 13
  injury severity score (ISS), 15t
    equation for, 15
  neurologic function examination of conscious patient, 14
  nonoperative methods of fracture care, 14
  skeleton stabilizing strategies, 14
  osteosynthesis, 14
  x-ray
    inappropriate use of, 13
    lateral, 14
POP. *See* Plaster-of-Paris
Positive end expiratory pressure (PEEP), 122
Posterior cruciate ligament (PCL), 123
Posterior dislocation of shoulder, 67
Posterior drawer test, 134
Primary bone healing, 30
Proximal humerus fractures, 66

Proximal interphalangeal (PIP), 96, 100-101
Proximal tibia and distal femur fractures, 124-128
Pseudoarthrosis, 5, 71
PTB. *See* Patellar tendon bearing cast
Pubic symphysis, inflammation of, 34*t*
PWB. *See* Partial-weight-bearing

Radial nerve injury, 69
Range of motion (ROM), 5, 63
Reduce, 5
ROM. *See* Range of motion
Rotator cuff injuries, 67
   abduction, 67
   external rotation, 67-68
   forward flexion, 67
Rotator cuff rupture, 68
Rotator cuff tear, 67, 68*t*

SAC. *See* Short arm cast
Sandwich splint, 71
Scaphoid, 91*f*, 93
Scapula, 63
   fractures, 66
Scar maturation, 27
Sciatic scoliosis, 175
Screwplate fixation, 14
Secondary bone healing, 30
Segond's fracture, 5, 124
SEX (situation, examination, x-ray), 7-8
Short arm cast (SAC), 5
Short leg cast (SLC), 5
Shoulder
   acromioclavicular separation, 63, 65*f*, 68*t*
     severe (grade III), 64*f*
   anterior dislocation, 67
     of humerus, 68*t*
   brachial plexus evaluation, 63
   clavicle fractures, 63, 64*f*, 65*f*, 66, 68*t*
   dislocations, 63, 67-68
     of humeral head, 65*f*
   fractures and dislocations about, 68*t*
   greater tuberosity fracture, 65*f*, 66
   posterior dislocations, 67
   proximal humerus fractures, 66
   range of motion, 63
   rotator cuff tear, 67, 68*t*
   scapula fractures, 66
   surgical neck fracture, 63, 65*f*, 68*t*
Siever's disease, 34*t*
Simple fracture, 5, 10, 11*f*
SITS. *See* Supraspinatus, infraspinatus, teres minor, subscapularis
Situation, evaluation, x-ray (SEX), 7
Skeletal traction, 54
Skeletal x-ray evaluation
   bone inspection
     fracture pattern, 10, 11*f*
     location of fracture, 9-10
   cataloging, 9
   describing apposition, 10
   describing location, 9-10
   examining joints, 10
   soft tissue inspection, 9
Skin, adult healing, 27, 28*f*
Skin traction, 53-54
   Buck's traction, 53, 54
SLC. *See* Short leg cast
Smith's fracture, 5
Soft tissue injuries, 95, 97, 100
   avulsion fracture, 100
   boutonniere deformity, 100
   of knee, 131*t*
   mallet finger, 100
   sprains, 97, 100
   strains, 97, 100
   tendon injuries, 100
Somatic pain, 43, 44*t*
Spine
   progressive loss of neurologic function, 23

Spine fractures, 163-165
  acute low back pain, 174-177
  anterior spinal artery syndrome, 165
  cervical spine fractures and dislocations, 166-171
  Frankel's grades below a transverse lesion, 165t
  hemisection of cord, 165
  spinal shock, 165
  thoracolumbar fractures, 171-174
  transverse myelopathy, 164
Spinal shock, 165
Spinal stenosis, 176t
Spiral fracture, 10, 11f, 69
Splint(s), 37, 38f, 39
  coaptation, 71
  definitive treatment, 37, 39, 40t
  limb positioning, 39
  sandwich, 71
  temporary, 37-38
  urgent immobilization, 37
Spondylolisthesis, 6, 176, 176t
Spondylosis, 5
Sprain(s), 6, 97, 100
  grading of, 8t
Steinmann pin, 55
Stockbroker's elbow, 77
Straddle fracture, 6
Straight-out traction, 53
Strains, 6, 97, 100
Stress fractures, 141, 143-144f
Subacromial bursa, 35
Subtalar dislocation, 157
Subtrochanteric fractures, 115
Supracondylar fractures, 124, 125
Supraspinatus, infraspinatus, teres minor, subscapularis (SITS), 67-68
Supraspinatus tendon, 35
Surgical neck fracture, 63, 65f, 68t
Suspension
  definition of, 53
  Thomas splint, 55, 56f
  Pearson attachment, 55, 56f
Swan-neck deformity, 97

Talus and calcaneus fractures and dislocations, 157-158
Temporary splints, 37
Tendinitis, 6, 33, 34
Tendon(s)
  Achilles', 34
  biceps, 34
  extensor, 34
  inflammation of, 34
  treating of, 34
Tendon healing time, 27, 31t
Tendon injuries, 100
Tendon repairs, 30
Tennis elbow, 77
Tenosynovitis, 6
Thomas ring splint with Pearson attachment, 55, 56f
Thomas splint, 55, 56f, 119
Thoracolumbar fractures, 171, 173-174
  Palmer's test, 174
Tib-fib fracture, 139
Tibial plateau fractures, 125
Tibial tubercle apophysitis, 34t
Tobramycin (antibiotic), 17
Torus fracture, 6
Traction
  axial, 67
  definition of, 53
  kit for skeletal, 55t
  lower limb traction, 55
  nontransfixing, 54
  skeletal, 54
  skin, 53
    Buck's traction, 53
    Steinmann pin, 55
    Thomas splint, 55
Trans-epiphyseal, 128f
Transfixing pins, 50
Transverse fracture, 10, 11f, 120
Transverse myelopathy, 164
Trapezium, 91f, 93
Trapezoid, 91f, 93
Traumatic amputations, compound fractures, 18, 21f
Triquetrum, 93
Trochanteric bursa, 35

Unstable spine, 169, 170f
Urgent immobilization, 37

Valgus, 6
Varus, 6
Venous tourniquet effect, 37
Visceral pain, 43, 44t
Volkmann's contracture, 84
Volkmann's ischemic contracture, 6, 78

WBAT. *See* Weight bearing as tolerated
Weber classification of fibula fractures, 147, 149t
Weight bearing as tolerated (WBAT), 6
Wrist injuries, 87
  accident-painful wrist, 89f
  intercarpal fractures and dislocations, 93
  lateral wrist x-ray, 91f
  nonarticular fracture of distal radius, 92f
  repetitive use painful conditions, 88t

X-ray(s)
  bone inspection
    fracture pattern, 10, 11f
    location of fracture, 9-10
  cataloging, 9
  describing apposition, 10
  elbow, 80f
  evaluating injury, 7-8
  examining joints, 10
  lateral wrist, 91f
  lateral cervical spine, 171, 172f
  pelvic, 104f, 106-107f
  polytrauma
    inappropriate use in, 13
    lateral, 14
  skeletal evaluation, 9-11
  soft tissue inspection, 9

Unstable spine, 169, 170f
Urgent immobilization, 37

Valgus, 6
Varus, 6
Venous tourniquet effect, 37
Visceral pain, 43, 44t
Volkmann's contracture, 84
Volkmann's ischemic contracture, 6, 78

WBAT. *See* Weight bearing as tolerated
Weber classification of fibula fractures, 147, 149t
Weight bearing as tolerated (WBAT), 6
Wrist injuries, 87
  accident-painful wrist, 89f
  intercarpal fractures and dislocations, 93
  lateral wrist x-ray, 91f
  nonarticular fracture of distal radius, 92f
  repetitive use painful conditions, 88t

X-ray(s)
  bone inspection
    fracture pattern, 10, 11f
    location of fracture, 9-10
  cataloging, 9
  describing apposition, 10
  elbow, 80f
  evaluating injury, 7-8
  examining joints, 10
  lateral wrist, 91f
  lateral cervical spine, 171, 172f
  pelvic, 104f, 106-107f
  polytrauma
    inappropriate use in, 13
    lateral, 14
  skeletal evaluation, 9-11
  soft tissue inspection, 9